New Mechanisms in Glucose Control

Anthony H. Barnett BSc, MD, FRCP

Professor of Medicine
Birmingham Heartlands Hospital
University of Birmingham and
Heart of England National Health Service Foundation Trust
Birmingham, UK

Jenny Grice BSc (Hons)

Medical Writer
Le Prioldy, Bieuzy les Eaux, France

WILEY-BLACKWELL

A John Wiley & Sons, Ltd., Publication

Contents

Preface

Whilst insulin was first isolated in 1921 and produced commercially by 1923, it was not until the mid 1950s that oral agents for type 2 diabetes came to the market, first sulphonylureas and then the first biguanide. We then waited another 30 years for the first alpha-glucosidase inhibitor, but since then there has been a veritable explosion in interest for new drugs in the diabetes market with a number now commercially available.

It is clear that the traditional agents remain important therapies, but they have their downside from the point of view of tolerability/side-effect problems. Moreover, they appear not to influence the natural history of the disease. The latter is an important issue given the progressive nature of type 2 diabetes and the need to achieve good glycaemic control to reduce the risk of devastating long-term vascular complications.

In the past few decades a revolution in our approach to treating type 2 diabetes has occurred following the recognition that the disease is caused by multiple defects. A range of new treatments are now available with differing mechanisms of action, and many more are in the pipeline, which will allow us to target this multifactorial disease more effectively than ever before.

The increasing requirement in the UK to move much of diabetes practice into the community requires a much more detailed knowledge of the condition by GPs and practice nurses. In this bespoke book, the authors aim to show how new mechanisms of glucose control and advances in treatments arising from this can be translated into primary care. The book will cover the epidemiology and pathogenesis of type 2 diabetes as well as provide an overview of current diabetes management including the pros and cons of traditional therapies. This will be followed by an in-depth discussion of the incretin system and the new drugs based on this approach – the incretin mimetics (glucagon-like peptide-1 (GLP-1) agonists) and dipeptidyl peptidase-4 (DPP-4) inhibitors. The authors will also review other drug classes in development as well as discussing the often observed resolution of type 2 diabetes that occurs after weight-loss surgery. Finally, they will consider effective approaches for diabetes care within that arena.

This book is particularly timely given the recent guidelines from the National Institute for Health and Clinical Excellence (NICE) on *Newer Agents for Blood Glucose Control in Type 2 Diabetes*, and is intended primarily for the multi-professional diabetes care team. It should, however, also be of interest to hospital specialists in training and other relevant staff. It is hoped that by increasing awareness of the expanding therapeutic options for type 2 diabetes and their mechanisms, we can better target the multitude of physiological defects that characterize the disease and customize treatment regimens to fit the individual needs of each patient.

Anthony H. Barnett
Birmingham

1 Epidemiology and Pathogenesis of Type 2 Diabetes

Throughout the world the increasing prevalence of diabetes is posing significant strains on already overburdened healthcare systems. Type 2 diabetes accounts for most of the projected increase, which reflects not only population growth and the demographics of an aging population, but also the increasing numbers of overweight and obese people who are at increased risk of diabetes.

The current prevalence of diabetes

Latest estimates from the International Diabetes Federation indicate that in 2010 the global prevalence of diabetes will be 285 million, representing 6.4% of the world's adult population, with a prediction that by 2030 the number of people with diabetes will have risen to 438 million (IDF, 2009).

In Europe, there is a wide variation in prevalence by country, but the total number of adults with diabetes in the region is expected to reach 55.2 million in 2010, accounting for 8.5% of the adult population (IDF, 2009). Estimates indicate that at least € 78 billion will be spent on healthcare for diabetes in the European Region in 2010, accounting for 28% of global expenditure (IDF, 2009).

In the United Kingdom (UK), there are now more than 2.6 million people with diabetes registered with general practices and more than 5.2 million registered as obese (Tables 1.1 and 1.2) (Diabetes UK, 2009). A recent analysis of UK data from The Health Improvement Network (THIN) database has shown a sharp jump in diabetes prevalence (Massó-González *et al.*, 2009). The study used data on 49 999 prevalent cases and 42 642 incident cases (1256 type 1 diabetes, 41 386 type 2 diabetes) of diabetes in UK patients aged 10 to 79 years in the THIN database. From 1996 to 2005, prevalence increased from 2.8% to 4.3%, while the incidence rose from 2.71 per 1000 person-years to 4.42 per 1000 person-years. The study also found that the proportion of patients newly diagnosed with type 2 diabetes who were obese increased from 46% to 56% during the decade, further highlighting the important role that obesity plays in the type 2 diabetes epidemic.

New Mechanisms in Glucose Control, First Edition. Anthony H. Barnett & Jenny Grice.
© 2011 Anthony H. Barnett & Jenny Grice. Published 2011 Blackwell Publishing Ltd.

Table 1.1 Prevalence of diabetes in people registered in UK general practice

	Diabetes		
Nation	Number of people with diabetes registered with GP practices in 2009	Diabetes prevalence in 2009 (%)	Increase in number of people with diabetes since 2008
England	2 213 138	5.1	124 803
Northern Ireland	65 066	4.5	4244
Wales	146 173	4.6	7185
Scotland	209 886	3.9	9217
UK total	2 634 263	4.0	145 449

Source: Diabetes UK (2009). Reproduced with permission.

   In the United States (US), recent predictions, which account for trends in risk factors such as obesity, the natural history of diabetes and the effects of treatments, suggest that the number of people with diagnosed and undiagnosed diabetes will double in the next 25 years from 23.7 million in 2009 to 44.1 million in 2034 (Huang *et al.*, 2009). Furthermore, the researchers predict that even if the prevalence of obesity remains stable, diabetes spending over the same period will nearly triple to US$336 billion.

Factors driving the type 2 diabetes epidemic

Age
The prevalence of type 2 diabetes increases with age and with more people living well into old age the likelihood of developing the disease is increased. However, increases in prevalence have been observed in younger age groups in association with the rising prevalence of childhood obesity and physical inactivity (Ehtisham, Barrett and Shaw, 2000; Fagot-Campagna, 2000). This is a

Table 1.2 Prevalence of obesity in people registered in UK general practice

	Obesity		
Nation	Number of people registered as obese with GP practices in 2009	Obesity prevalence in 2009 (%)	Increase in number of people registered as obese since 2008
England	4 389 964	9.9	260 660
Northern Ireland	165 956	11.27	4085
Wales	305 923	9.7	5442
Scotland	375 649	7.0	22 476
UK total	5 237 492	8.1	292 663

Source: Diabetes UK (2009). Reproduced with permission.

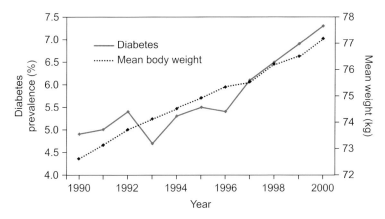

Figure 1.1 The growing epidemic of type 2 diabetes in relation to obesity (Mokdad *et al.*, 2000). Data from *Diabetes Care* 2000; 23:1278–1283, Copyright 2000 American Diabetes Association.

worrying finding given that the risk of complications increases with duration of disease.

Overweight and obesity

More and more of the world's population is being exposed to the dietary habits and sedentary lifestyles of the developed nations. The increase in calorie intake, mainly derived from carbohydrates and animal fat, with a decrease in physical activity, has led to excessive obesity and increasing resistance to insulin action. Type 2 diabetes is strongly associated with overweight and obesity (Figure 1.1) (Mokdad *et al.*, 2000), and a high proportion of people with type 2 diabetes are overweight or obese at the time of diagnosis, which may reach up to 80% in some populations (Hedley *et al.*, 2004).

In the UK, rates of obesity have dramatically increased in the past two decades. The ongoing Health Survey for England highlights the increasing trend. In 1993, 13% of men and 16% of women were estimated to be obese (body mass index (BMI) $>30 \text{ kg/m}^2$) (DoH, 1994). Just over a decade later the proportion of men and women classed as obese had increased to 24% for both sexes (DoH, 2004). The Foresight report 'Tackling Obesities: Future Choices', which was commissioned by the UK Government, has estimated that if no action is taken, 60% of men, 50% of women and 25% of under-20 year olds will be obese by 2050 based on current trends (Foresight, 2007).

Socioeconomic class

The prevalence of diabetes appears to be higher amongst low socioeconomic groups, with a 36% higher prevalence noted amongst men living in the most deprived areas of England and Wales compared with those living in the most affluent areas. For women the prevalence amongst those living in the most deprived areas is 80% higher than amongst those living in the least deprived parts. Interestingly, the reverse situation is found in developing countries

(Mohan *et al.*, 2001).The tendency for the increased prevalence of type 2 diabetes to be concentrated in lower socioeconomic groups in developed countries and higher socioeconomic groups in developing countries probably reflects the adoption of a healthier lifestyle by better educated people in developed countries, while it is generally the affluent in developing countries who enjoy a high calorie intake and low level of physical activity.

Ethnicity

Certain ethnic minorities (e.g. individuals originating from the Indian subcontinent, Pima Indians, Mexican Americans, and African Americans) appear to have an increased susceptibility to develop insulin resistance when meeting certain environmental factors including obesity and a sedentary lifestyle and are more prone to type 2 diabetes than Caucasians (Barnett *et al.*, 2006). These populations may have an increased genetic susceptibility to lay down intra-abdominal fat, particularly when encountering a Western style of living.

In the UK, the risk of type 2 diabetes is increased four- to sixfold in South Asians compared with Caucasians (Barnett *et al.*, 2006). The age at presentation is also significantly younger (UKPDS, 1994). As duration of diabetes is one of the strongest risk factors for complications, this places this population at particular risk.

Pathogenesis of type 2 diabetes

Type 2 diabetes is characterized by three main defects: peripheral insulin resistance (decreased glucose uptake in muscle, fat and the liver), excess hepatic glucose output, and a pancreatic beta-cell insulin-secretory deficit. The development of the condition is a gradual process, however, and in most individuals, insulin resistance is the first defect to occur (Haffner *et al.*, 2000). Both genetic and environmental factors play a role in the pathogenesis of type 2 diabetes, but one of the most common causes of insulin resistance is obesity, particularly abdominal obesity.

Insulin resistance precedes abnormalities in insulin secretion by several years because pancreatic beta cells are initially able to compensate for insulin resistance by increasing insulin secretion sufficiently to maintain normal blood glucose levels. Eventually, the beta cells become exhausted, however, and can no longer produce enough insulin.

Following a meal, insulin is produced in two phases. First-phase insulin secretion is released rapidly after a meal, and it is this response that is lost very early in type 2 diabetes. When the first-phase insulin response fails, plasma glucose levels rise sharply after a meal producing postprandial hyperglycaemia. Initially, this precipitates an increased stimulation of second-phase insulin release, but eventually this too will be blunted and fasting hyperglycaemia will also result.

The results of the United Kingdom Prospective Diabetes Study (UKPDS) demonstrated that beta-cell function is already reduced at the time of diagnosis of type 2 diabetes and continues to deteriorate despite treatment (UKPDS 33, 1998). The mechanisms responsible for the progressive loss of beta-cell function are still unclear, although a number of hypotheses exist. Some data suggest that genetic abnormalities may result in increased apoptosis and decreased regeneration of beta cells. Over-stimulation of the beta cells in the early years of insulin resistance may lead to increased rates of beta-cell death. Another possibility is that prolonged hyperglycaemia could lead to beta-cell loss or dysfunction through glucotoxicity (Kaiser, Leibowitz and Nesher, 2003) or lipotoxicity mechanisms (Smiley, 2003).

In the past decade, research on the incretin hormones has increased our understanding of the pathogenesis of type 2 diabetes. The predominant incretin hormone is glucagon-like peptide-1 (GLP-1), which has a number of functions including: stimulation of glucose-dependent insulin secretion, suppression of glucagon secretion, slowing of gastric emptying, reduction of food intake, and improved insulin sensitivity. Secretion of GLP-1 is lower than normal in patients with type 2 diabetes (Vilsbøll *et al.*, 2001), and increasing GLP-1 decreases hyperglycaemia, which suggests that the hormone may contribute to the pathogenesis of the disease (Drucker, 2003). As a result of research in this area, most new treatments for type 2 diabetes are being designed based on an understanding of the full pathophysiology of diabetes targeting all major defects.

References

Barnett AH, Dixon AN, Bellary S, *et al.* (2006) Type 2 diabetes and cardiovascular risk in the UK South Asian community. *Diabetologia*; 49:2234–2246.

Department of Health (DoH). Health Survey for England 1994: cardiovascular disease and associated risk factors. Available from: http://www.dh.gov.uk/en/Publicationsandstatistics/PublishedSurvey/HealthSurveyForEngland/Healthsurveyresults/DH_4001552. Last accessed February 2010.

Department of Health (DoH). Health Survey for England 2004: Health of ethnic minorities. Available from: http://www.ic.nhs.uk/statistics-and-data-collections/health-and-lifestyles-related-surveys/health-survey-for-england/health-survey-for-england-2004:-health-of-ethnic-minorities–full-report. Last accessed February 2010.

Diabetes UK [News release, 2 October 2009]. Diabetes and obesity rates soar. Available from: http://www.diabetes.org.uk/About_us/News_Landing_Page/Diabetes-and-obesity-rates-soar. Last accessed February 2010.

Drucker DJ. (2003) Glucagon-like peptides: regulators of cell proliferation, differentiation, and apoptosis. *Mol Endocrinol*; 17:161–171.

Ehtisham S, Barrett TG, Shaw NJ. (2000) Type 2 diabetes mellitus in UK children – an emerging problem. *Diabet Med*; 17:867–871.

Fagot-Campagna A. (2000) Emergence of type 2 diabetes mellitus in children: epidemiological evidence. *J Pediatr Endocrinol Metab*; 13 (Suppl 6):1395–1402.

Foresight (2007) Tackling Obesities: Future Choices – Modelling Future Trends in Obesity & Their Impact on Health. Available from: http://www.foresight.gov.uk/Obesity/14.pdf. Last accessed February 2010.

Haffner SM, Mykkanen L, Festa A, *et al.* (2000) Insulin-resistant prediabetic subjects have more atherogenic risk factors than insulin-sensitive prediabetic subjects: implications for preventing coronary heart disease during the prediabetic state. *Circulation*; 101:975–980.

Hedley AA, Ogden CL, Johnson CL, *et al.* (2004) Prevalence of overweight and obesity among US children, adolescents, and adults, 1999–2002. *JAMA*; 291:2847–2850.

Huang ES, Basu A, O'Grady M, Capretta JC. (2009) Projecting the future diabetes population size and related costs for the U.S. *Diabetes Care*; 32:2225–2229.

International Diabetes Federation (2009) IDF Diabetes Atlas, 4th Edition. Available from: http://www.diabetesatlas.org/content/europe. Last accessed December 2009.

Kaiser N, Leibowitz G, Nesher R. (2003) Glucotoxicity and beta-cell failure in type 2 diabetes mellitus. *J Pediatr Endocrinol Metab*; 16:5–22.

Massó-González EL, Johansson S, Wallander M-A, García-Rodríguez LA. Trends in the prevalence and incidence of diabetes in the UK – 1996 to 2005. *J Epidemiol Community Health*; doi:10.1136/jech.2008.080382.

Mohan V, Shanthirani S, Deepa R, *et al.* (2001) Intra-urban differences in the prevalence of the metabolic syndrome in southern India – the Chennai Urban Population Study (CUPS No. 4). *Diabet Med*; 18:280–287.

Mokdad AH, Ford ES, Bowman BA, *et al.* (2000) Diabetes trends in the US: 1990–1998. *Diabetes Care*; 23:1278–1283.

Smiley T. (2003) The role of declining beta cell function in the progression of type 2 diabetes: implications for outcomes and pharmacological management. *Can J Diabetes*; 27:277–286.

UK Prospective Diabetes Study (UKPDS) Group (1994) UK Prospective Diabetes Study XII: Differences between Asian, Afro-Caribbean and white Caucasian type 2 diabetic patients at diagnosis of diabetes. *Diabet Med*; 11:670–677.

UK Prospective Diabetes Study (UKPDS) Group (1998) Intensive blood-glucose control with sulphonylureas or insulin compared with conventional treatment and risk of complications in patients with type 2 diabetes (UKPDS 33). *Lancet*; 352:854–865.

Vilsbøll T, Krarup T, Deacon CF, *et al.* (2001) Reduced postprandial concentrations of intact biologically active glucagon-like peptide 1 in type 2 diabetic patients. *Diabetes*; 50:609–613.

2 Overview of Current Diabetes Management

Following the sharp increase in diabetes prevalence that has occurred over the last few decades, 2.3 million people in England aged 17 years or over (NHS Information Centre, 2010) and 228 thousand people in Scotland (Scottish Diabetes Survey, 2009) were recorded on GP diabetes registers as of March 2010. With such a large population, routine clinical care for many of these patients is now managed mainly in primary care. Treatment should be aimed at alleviating symptoms and minimizing the risk of long-term complications with the overall aim of enabling people with diabetes to achieve a quality of life and life expectancy similar to that of the general population. Although this publication focuses on new mechanisms for glucose control, cardiovascular disease is the leading cause of morbidity and mortality in patients with type 2 diabetes, and management of diabetes needs to be multifactorial aiming to reduce complications by careful control of blood glucose as well as other cardiovascular risk factors.

Recommended targets for glycaemic control

Setting goals appropriate for the individual

People with type 2 diabetes form a diverse group varying significantly in terms of risk factors, disease duration, age, glycaemic control, comorbid conditions, prescribed antidiabetes treatment, and commitment to self-management. Furthermore, as type 2 diabetes is characterized by insulin resistance and ongoing decline in pancreatic beta-cell function, glucose levels are likely to worsen over time (UKPDS 16, 1995). Management must therefore be dynamic and tailored to the individual needs and circumstances of each patient.

Blood glucose levels as close to the normal range should be the goal if this can be achieved safely, but targets may often have to be a compromise between what is theoretically achievable and what is best for the individual patient. For example, a young patient diagnosed with diabetes but otherwise healthy would normally have a lower glycaemic target than an elderly patient with comorbidities receiving several concomitant medications.

Glycaemic control: how low should we go?

In 2010, the UK National Institute for Health and Clinical Excellence (NICE) advisory committee for the Quality and Outcomes Framework (QOF) recommended that the HbA_{1c} target for people with type 2 diabetes in general be raised from 7.0% (53 mmol/mol) to 7.5% (59 mmol/mol) (NICE, 2010a). This was in response to concern that to achieve an average practice target HbA_{1c} of 7.0% (53 mmol/mol), physicians would need to aim for a level lower than this in individual patients. The publication of the large Action to Control Cardiovascular Risk in Diabetes (ACCORD), Action in Diabetes and Vascular Disease: Preterax and Diamicron Modified Release Controlled Evaluation (ADVANCE), and Veterans Affairs Diabetes Trial (VADT) studies, which investigated the effects of rigorous metabolic control on the prevalence of cardiovascular outcomes in type 2 diabetes, has raised questions about whether tight glucose control strategies are therapeutically desirable (Lehman and Krumholz, 2009; Yudkin, 2008).

The ACCORD trial was stopped prematurely in 2008 due to increased mortality in the intensive therapy group (ACCORD, 2008), and the ADVANCE (ADVANCE, 2008) and VADT (Duckworth *et al.*, 2009) trials showed no benefit on cardiovascular outcomes and mortality. The overall conclusion from the three studies was that HbA_{1c} values less than 7.0% (53 mmol/mol) (less than 6% (42 mmol/mol) in ACCORD) did not produce a statistically significant reduction in macrovascular events, but did produce a marked increase in hypoglycaemia (Figure 2.1).

The study population in the ACCORD, ADVANCE and VADT trials was predominantly elderly with advanced diabetes and known cardiovascular disease or multiple risk factors, suggesting the presence of established atherosclerosis. It has been suggested that the increase in mortality in ACCORD may have been related to the intensive treatment strategies used in this population to rapidly reduce HbA_{1c} by at least 2 percentage points and not the level of HbA_{1c} achieved (Skyler *et al.*, 2009). In support of this, the

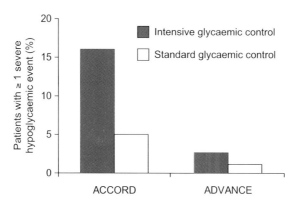

Figure 2.1 Absolute rates of severe hypoglycaemia (percentage of patients affected during the trial) in the two glucose arms of the ACCORD and ADVANCE trials (ACCORD, 2008; ADVANCE, 2008).

ADVANCE trial, which reduced levels less aggressively than ACCORD, achieved a similar median HbA$_{1c}$ in its intensive arm, but with no increased mortality (ADVANCE, 2008).

The controversy continues as not all studies have replicated the findings of ACCORD, ADVANCE and VADT. The UKPDS-80 trial, a follow-up of the original UKPDS, found that intensive glycaemic control was beneficial when initiated in newly diagnosed patients, with a continued reduction in risk of microvascular complications and reductions in risk for myocardial infarction and death from any cause that emerged during 10 years of post-trial follow-up (Holman *et al.*, 2008). Contrasting findings have also been reported in a recent meta-analysis of five large randomized clinical trials, including UKPDS, ADVANCE, VADT, ACCORD, and the PROspective pioglitAzone Clinical Trial in macroVascular Events (PROactive) (Ray *et al.*, 2009). Although there was no effect on stroke or all-cause mortality, a 17% reduction in myocardial infarction and a 15% reduction in the risk of coronary heart disease events were reported.

Current consensus on glycaemic control targets

The general consensus is that the ACCORD findings should not deter healthcare providers from helping patients achieve recommended glycaemic targets (Skyler *et al.*, 2009). Rather, the results further illustrate the need to tailor HbA$_{1c}$ targets and treatments to individual patients. The ACCORD results show that intensive treatment of hyperglycaemia may not be beneficial in high-risk patients with a long history of type 2 diabetes. Long-term UKPDS results show there are benefits of intensive care at an early stage of the disease. The potential risks of intensive glycaemic control may therefore outweigh its benefits in some patients, such as those with a very long duration of diabetes, known history of severe hypoglycaemia, advanced atherosclerosis, and advanced age/frailty. NICE cautions against intensive efforts to get below current treatment targets recognizing that successful control of diabetes cannot be measured by setting HbA$_{1c}$ targets that are independent of the patient and their personal health factors and lifestyle.

Pros and cons of existing non-insulin antidiabetes therapies

Despite the value of diet and lifestyle measures, most patients with type 2 diabetes will also require pharmacotherapy to achieve glycaemic goals. There are now eight classes of non-insulin antidiabetes therapies for treating type 2 diabetes (metformin, sulphonylureas, meglitinides, thiazolidinediones, alpha-glucosidase inhibitors, amylin analogues, glucagon-like peptide-1 (GLP-1) receptor agonists, and dipeptidyl peptidase 4 (DPP-4) inhibitors. These agents act at different sites in the body to improve insulin secretion or improve insulin action (Table 2.1). Antidiabetes agents can be used alone or in combination to provide therapy for type 2 diabetes. A number of factors need to be considered when deciding on the choice of drug or drug combination to use in an individual (Table 2.2).

Table 2.1　Classes of non-insulin antidiabetes therapies for the treatment of type 2 diabetes

Antidiabetes therapy	Primary mechanism of action
Metformin	Inhibition of hepatic gluconeogenesis and increase in hepatic insulin sensitivity
Sulphonylureas	Stimulation of insulin secretion
Meglitinides	Stimulation of insulin secretion
Thiazolidinediones	Increase in muscle, liver and adipose tissue insulin sensitivity
Alpha-glucosidase inhibitors	Delay in glucose absorption
Amylin analogue	Inhibition of gastric emptying and glucagon release, reduces food intake
GLP-1 receptor agonists	Stimulation of glucose-dependent insulin secretion and inhibition of glucagon release
DPP-4 inhibitors	Stimulation of glucose-dependent insulin secretion and inhibition of glucagon release via increase in endogenous GLP-1

Metformin

Metformin is recognized as the first-line treatment for type 2 diabetes in patients not achieving adequate glycaemic control with diet and lifestyle interventions, particularly in individuals who are overweight, and can also be prescribed as adjunct therapy to virtually every other antidiabetes agent

Table 2.2　Factors influencing target HbA_{1c} goal and choice of antidiabetes therapy

- Severity of hyperglycaemia
- Risk of hypoglycaemia
- Weight/body mass index
- Stage of disease
  - recently diagnosed
  - long duration
- Cardiovascular risk profile
- Medical conditions
  - renal function
  - oedema
  - heart failure
  - osteoporosis
- Medication side-effects
- Occupation
  - driving/flying/working at heights
- Practical issues
  - eyesight/manual dexterity/cognitive function
  - likely adherence to frequency of dosing
- Patient preference
- Social e.g. patient living alone

currently available (Nathan *et al.*, 2006; NICE 2008; NICE, 2009). Metformin has no direct effects on beta cells, but reduces blood glucose levels by suppressing hepatic glucose production, increasing the sensitivity of muscle cells to insulin, and decreasing absorption of glucose from the gastrointestinal tract (Strack, 2008).

Benefits	Disadvantages
• HbA$_{1c}$ reductions of up to 1.5% as monotherapy • No weight gain • Low risk of hypoglycaemia • Non-glycaemic benefits include improvements in atherogenic lipid profiles and reduction in cardiovascular event rates and mortality (UKPDS 34, 1998)	• Gastrointestinal side-effects common • Very rare risk of lactic acidosis when renal clearance limited (Bodmer *et al.*, 2008)

Sulphonylureas

For people in whom metformin is contraindicated or not tolerated, guidelines generally recommend a sulphonylurea as a suitable first-line alternative if the person is not overweight (NICE, 2009). A sulphonylurea is also generally added as second-line therapy when blood glucose control remains or becomes inadequate with metformin. The sulphonylureas reduce blood glucose levels by increasing insulin secretion from beta cells and therefore they work only in patients who have sufficient remaining beta-cell function.

Benefits	Disadvantages
• Rapid onset of action and almost immediate effects on blood glucose • HbA$_{1c}$ reductions of up to 1.5% as monotherapy	• Weight gain common • Risk of hypoglycaemia especially with long-acting agents, which limits their use particularly in the elderly (Zammit and Frier, 2005) • Coadministration with drugs that inhibit hepatic metabolism of sulphonylureas may further increase hypoglycaemia risk (Campbell, 2009)

Meglitinides

The meglitinides have a mode of action that is similar to that of the sulphonylureas, but bind to a different receptor on the beta-cell potassium channel. They were developed to have a rapid onset of action and short metabolic half-life so as to preferentially stimulate insulin secretion in the postprandial state. As a result, they are most beneficial when control of fasting plasma glucose is good but HbA$_{1c}$ levels are high. The meglitinides are taken 15–30 minutes before the start of a meal and if a meal is missed the medication should not be taken. For this reason they are generally only recommended for individuals with erratic lifestyles (NICE, 2009).

Benefits	Disadvantages
• Rapid onset of action • Repaglinide associated with HbA$_{1c}$ reduction of up to 1.5% as monotherapy, nateglinide slightly less	• Weight gain common • Hypoglycaemia, although less than with sulphonylureas, but risk increased with drug interactions • Multiple daily dosing required

Thiazolidinediones

The thiazolidinediones (TZDs) work primarily by activating the nuclear transcription factor peroxisome proliferator-activated receptor gamma (PPAR-γ), which is involved in the transcription of genes that regulate glucose and fat metabolism. The most prominent effect of TZDs is to enhance insulin sensitivity and subsequent glucose uptake by skeletal muscle, liver and adipose cells (Mudaliar *et al.*, 2001), which results in a reduction in insulin concentrations (Hoffmann and Spengler, 1997). The TZDs complement existing treatment approaches for type 2 diabetes. Although the TZDs and metformin effectively increase sensitivity to insulin, they have different target organs – metformin exerting most of its glycaemic effect by decreasing hepatic glucose production and the TZDs by enhancing insulin sensitivity primarily in muscle and adipose tissue (Barnett, 2009). NICE has temporarily withdrawn its recommendations on the use of rosiglitazone following the decision of the European Medicines Agency (EMA) to suspend the marketing authorization for this agent across the European Union after concluding that the benefits of rosiglitazone no longer outweigh its risks (NICE, 2010b). Pioglitazone is therefore the only agent in this class currently available.

Benefits	Disadvantages
• HbA$_{1c}$ reductions of up to 1.5% as monotherapy • Low risk of hypoglycaemia • Preservation of markers of beta-cell function (Leiter, 2005) • Sustained long-term glycaemic control (Kahn *et al.*, 2006) • Non-glycaemic benefits include improvements in atherogenic lipid profiles and inflammatory markers • Pioglitazone demonstrated reductions in atheroma volume (Nissen *et al.*, 2008) and benefits on cardiovascular outcomes (Dormandy *et al.*, 2005)	• Slow onset of action • Weight gain common • Fluid retention may lead to oedema and new or worsening heart failure • Rosiglitazone not recommended in patients with ischaemic heart disease (Nissen and Wolski, 2007; Rosen, 2007) • Increased risk of distal bone fracture (Meier *et al.*, 2008; Monami *et al.*, 2008)

Alpha-glucosidase inhibitors

The primary mechanism of action of the alpha-glucosidase inhibitors is to delay the digestion of carbohydrates in the small intestine and therefore their main use is in controlling postprandial plasma glucose (van de Laar, 2008). The alpha-glucosidase inhibitors are not dependent on adequate beta-cell function and their effectiveness does not decrease over time. The three available agents: acarbose, miglitol, and voglibose can be used as monotherapy alongside appropriate diet and exercise regimens, or added to other medications.

Benefits	Disadvantages
• HbA$_{1c}$ reductions of 0.5–0.8% as monotherapy • Low risk of hypoglycaemia • No weight gain • Acarbose has demonstrated benefits on cardiovascular outcomes beyond glycaemic control (Chiasson *et al.*, 2002)	• Gastrointestinal side-effects common, particularly flatulence, diarrhoea and bloating (Hanefeld, 2007) • Must be taken with meals containing digestible carbohydrates

Amylin analogues (not licensed in Europe)

Amylin is secreted by the beta cells in response to increased glucose levels and effects glucose control through several mechanisms, including slowed gastric emptying, regulation of postprandial glucagon, and reduction of food intake (Ryan *et al.*, 2005). Amylin is reduced in people with type 2 diabetes, which has led to the development of a synthetic analogue known as pramlintide. This agent is indicated in patients with type 2 diabetes as an adjunct to meal-time insulin therapy, with or without a concurrent sulphonylurea and/or metformin.

Benefits	Disadvantages
• HbA$_{1c}$ reductions of 0.3–0.6% • Reduction in body weight (independent of nausea) (Ryan *et al.*, 2005) • Beta-cell function not required for glucose-lowering effect so can be used in a population with advanced disease	• Nausea common • High risk of hypoglycaemia when beginning therapy • Pramlintide and insulin must be given as two separate injections • Careful selection of patients required because of the risk of hypoglycaemia, complexity of dosing and administration

Why are new drugs needed for the treatment of type 2 diabetes?

Type 2 diabetes is a chronic disease affecting an ever increasing number of people, yet while available agents may initially be effective at achieving recommended levels of glycaemic control, long-term efficacy is difficult to achieve without regular adjustment and combination therapy. In addition, with the possible exception of the TZDs, established agents have little effect on the underlying cause of disease progression, that is, the declining function of pancreatic beta cells. The increased risk for hypoglycaemia and the weight gain associated with several therapies also represent major barriers to optimal glycaemic control. It is becoming increasingly recognized that it is important to bear in mind not just by how much a drug lowers blood glucose, but also the mechanisms by which this occurs. In addition to lowering blood glucose, new classes of agent for diabetes control are therefore focusing on the main unmet needs in diabetes management: better tolerability, prolonged efficacy and the potential to act on the underlying cause of the disease.

References

The Action to Control Cardiovascular Risk in Diabetes (ACCORD) Study Group (2008) Effects of intensive glucose lowering in type 2 diabetes. *N Engl J Med*; 358:2545–2549.

The ADVANCE Collaborative Group (2008) Intensive blood glucose control and vascular outcomes in patients with type 2 diabetes. *N Engl J Med*; 358:2560–2572.

Barnett AH. (2009) Redefining the role of thiazolidinediones in the management of type 2 diabetes. *Vasc Health Risk Manag*; 5:141–51.

Bodmer M, Meier C, Krähenbühl S, *et al.* (2008) Metformin, sulfonylureas, or other antidiabetes drugs and the risk of lactic acidosis or hypoglycemia: a nested case-control analysis. *Diabetes Care*; 31:2086–2091.

Campbell IW. (2009) Sulfonylureas and hypoglycemia. *Diabetic Hypoglycemia*; 2:3–10.

Chiasson JL, Josse RG, Gomis R, *et al.*; STOP-NIDDM Trial Research Group (2002) Acarbose for prevention of type 2 diabetes mellitus: the STOP-NIDDM randomised trial. *Lancet*; 359:2072–2077.

Dormandy JA, Charbonnel B, Eckland DJ, *et al.*; PROactive investigators (2005) Secondary prevention of macrovascular events in patients with type 2 diabetes in the PROactive Study (PROspective pioglitAzone Clinical Trial In macroVascular Events): a randomised controlled trial. *Lancet*; 366:1279–1289.

Duckworth W, Abraira C, Moritz T, *et al*; VADT Investigators (2009) Glucose control and vascular complications in veterans with type 2 diabetes. *N Engl J Med*; 360:129–139.

Hanefeld M. (2007) Cardiovascular benefits and safety profile of acarbose therapy in prediabetes and established type 2 diabetes. *Cardiovasc Diabetol*; 6:20.

Hoffmann J, Spengler M. (1997) Efficacy of 24-week monotherapy with acarbose, metformin, or placebo in dietary-treated NIDDM patients: the Essen-II Study. *Am J Med*; 103:483–490.

Holman RR, Paul SK, Bethel MA, *et al.* (2008) 10-year follow-up of intensive glucose control in type 2 diabetes. *N Engl J Med*; 359:1577–1589.

Kahn SE, Haffner SM, Heise MA, *et al.*; ADOPT Study Group (2006) Glycemic durability of rosiglitazone, metformin, or glyburide monotherapy. *N Engl J Med*; 355:2427–2443.

Lehman R, Krumholz HM. (2009) Tight control of blood glucose in long standing type 2 diabetes. *BMJ*; 338:b800.

Leiter LA. (2005) Beta-cell preservation: a potential role for thiazolidinediones to improve clinical care in type 2 diabetes. *Diabet Med*; 22:963–972.

Meier C, Kraenzlin ME, Bodmer M, *et al.* (2008) Use of thiazolidinediones and fracture risk. *Arch Intern Med*; 168:820–825.

Monami M, Cresci B, Colombini A, *et al.* (2008) Bone fractures and hypoglycemic treatment in type 2 diabetic patients: a case-control study. *Diabetes Care*; 31:199–203.

Mudaliar S, Henry RR. (2001) New oral therapies for type 2 diabetes mellitus: the glitazones or insulin sensitizers. *Annu Rev Med*; 52:239–257.

Nathan DM, Buse JB, Davidson MB, *et al.* (2006) Management of hyperglycaemia in type 2 diabetes: a consensus algorithm for the initiation and adjustment of therapy. *Diabetologia*; 49:1711–1721.

National Health Service. Quality and Outcomes Framework. Online GP practice results database. Available from: http://www.ic.nhs.uk/webfiles/QOF/2009-10/Prevalence%20tables/QOF0910_National_Prevalence.xls. Last accessed December 2010.

National Institute for Health and Clinical Excellence (NICE) (2008) Type 2 diabetes: the management of type 2 diabetes (update). Available from: http://www.nice.org.uk/CG66. Last accessed February 2010.

National Institute for Health and Clinical Excellence (NICE) (2009) Type 2 diabetes: newer agents for blood glucose control. NICE short clinical guidelines 87. Available from: http://www.nice.org.uk/nicemedia/pdf/CG87NICEGuideline.pdf. Last accessed February 2010.

National Institute for Health and Clinical Excellence (NICE) (2010a) NICE indicator guidance for QOF. Available from: http://www.nice.org.uk/nicemedia/live/13081/50073/50073.pdf. Last accessed December 2010.

National Institute for Health and Clinical Excellence (NICE) (2010b) The European Medicines Agency (EMA) and rosiglitazone. Available from: http://guidance.nice.org.uk/CG66. Last accessed December 2010.

Nissen SE, Wolski K. (2007) Effect of rosiglitazone on the risk of myocardial infarction and death from cardiovascular causes. *N Engl J Med*; 356:2457–2471.

Nissen SE, Nicholls SJ, Wolski K, *et al.*; PERISCOPE Investigators (2008) Comparison of pioglitazone vs glimepiride on progression of coronary atherosclerosis in patients with type 2 diabetes: the PERISCOPE randomized controlled trial. *JAMA*; 299:1561–1573.

Ray KK, Seshasai SR, Wijesuriya S, *et al.* (2009) Effect of intensive control of glucose on cardiovascular outcomes and death in patients with diabetes mellitus: a meta-analysis of randomized controlled trials. *Lancet*; 373:1765–1772.

Rosen CJ. (2007) The rosiglitazone story – lessons from an FDA Advisory Committee meeting. *N Engl J Med*; 357:844–846.

Ryan GJ, Jobe LJ, Martin R. (2005) Pramlintide in the treatment of type 1 and type 2 diabetes mellitus. *Clin Ther*; 27:1500–1512.

Scottish Diabetes Survey Monitoring Group (2009) Scottish Diabetes Survey 2009. Available from: http://www.diabetesinscotland.org.uk/Publications/Scottish%20Diabetes%20Survey%202009.pdf. Last accessed December 2010.

Skyler JS, Bergenstal R, Bonow RO, *et al.*; American Diabetes Association; American College of Cardiology Foundation; American Heart Association (2009) Intensive glycemic control and the prevention of cardiovascular events: implications of the ACCORD, ADVANCE, and VA Diabetes Trials: a position statement of the American Diabetes Association and a Scientific Statement of the American College of Cardiology Foundation and the American Heart Association. *J Am Coll Cardiol*; 53:298–304.

Strack T. (2008) Metformin: a review. *Drugs Today (Barc)*; 44:303–314.

UK Prospective Diabetes Study 16 (UKPDS 16) (1995) Overview of 6 years' therapy of type II diabetes: a progressive disease. *UKPDS Group.* Diabetes; 44:1249–1258.

UK Prospective Diabetes Study 34 (UKPDS 34) (1998) Effect of intensive blood-glucose control with metformin on complications in overweight patients with type 2 diabetes. UKPDS Group. *Lancet*; 352:854–865.

van de Laar FA. (2008) Alpha-glucosidase inhibitors in the early treatment of type 2 diabetes. *Vasc Health Risk Manag*; 4:1189–1195.

Yudkin JS. (2008) Very tight glucose control – may be high risk, low benefit. *BMJ*; 336:683.

Zammitt NN, Frier BM. (2005) Hypoglycemia in type 2 diabetes: pathophysiology, frequency, and effects of different treatment modalities. *Diabetes Care*; 28:2948–2961.

3 The Incretin System

The incretin system has come to the forefront of attention in the past decade as a potential source of new therapies for type 2 diabetes, but the concept initially surfaced nearly half a century ago following the observation that orally administered glucose stimulates a far greater release of insulin than the same amount of glucose delivered by injection (Elrick *et al.*, 1964). Research focused on discovering the signal that triggered the gastrointestinal tract to release insulin whenever food is consumed and found that two hormones are responsible for this effect in humans: glucagon-like peptide-1 (GLP-1) and glucose-dependent insulinotropic polypeptide (GIP) – the incretin hormones.

It is now known that following secretion from the gastrointestinal tract during food intake the incretin hormones bind to receptors on beta cells of the pancreas, thereby stimulating insulin secretion in response to glucose absorption (Ahrén, 2003). In healthy individuals, the incretin effect is thought to be responsible for 50–70% of the insulin response to oral glucose, but secretion is lower than normal in patients with type 2 diabetes suggesting that decreased levels are involved in the pathogenesis of the disease (Nauck *et al.*, 1986; Vilsbøll *et al.*, 2001). This is further supported by the fact that increasing GLP-1 levels decreases hyperglycaemia (Drucker, 2003).

GLP-1 and GIP stimulate insulin secretion in a glucose-dependent manner so that insulin is secreted only when blood glucose is elevated. GIP is not active in patients with type 2 diabetes, however, and the focus of research has therefore been on GLP-1, which has multiple blood glucose-lowering effects (Figure 3.1). In addition to glucose-dependent insulin secretion, GLP-1 regulates glucose homeostasis via inhibition of glucagon secretion (thereby reducing liver glucose output) and gastric emptying. The latter slows the absorption of carbohydrate and the resulting rise in blood glucose after a meal. GLP-1 also appears to curb appetite leading to long-term control of body weight. Animal studies have shown that GLP-1 may promote regeneration of pancreatic beta cells and prevent apoptosis, improving the survival of existing beta cells (Drucker, 2003).

The incretin hormones affect a number of important pathophysiological mechanisms that are not currently targeted by conventional therapies for type

New Mechanisms in Glucose Control, First Edition. Anthony H. Barnett & Jenny Grice.
© 2011 Anthony H. Barnett & Jenny Grice. Published 2011 Blackwell Publishing Ltd.

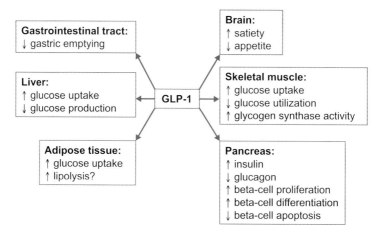

Figure 3.1 The glucose-lowering actions of GLP-1 in pancreatic and extrapancreatic tissue. Reproduced from Grossman (2009) with permission from Pharmacotherapy.

2 diabetes, including beta-cell dysfunction and altered glucagon secretion by the alpha cells. The native peptides are, however, rapidly removed from the circulation by the enzyme dipeptidyl peptidase-4 (DPP-4) as well as by renal clearance (Deacon *et al.*, 1995). Significant research has therefore focused on producing incretin-based therapies with longer half-lives using two different approaches. The first was to develop GLP-1 receptor agonists that are resistant to DPP-4 – the incretin mimetics. The two products in this category are exenatide and liraglutide. Both are peptides and therefore need to be injected, but this also allows GLP-1 concentrations to be increased above endogenous levels with potentially greater treatment effects. The second approach was to develop agents that inhibit DPP-4 – the DPP-4 inhibitors or incretin enhancers. These agents can be administered orally, but are dependent on endogenous levels of GLP-1 for their action.

References

Ahrén B. (2003) Gut peptides and type 2 diabetes mellitus treatment. *Curr Diab Rep*; 3:365–372.

Deacon CF, Nauck MA, Toft-Nielsen M, *et al.* (1995) Both subcutaneously and intravenously administered glucagon-like peptide 1 are rapidly degraded from the NH2-terminus in type II diabetic patients and in healthy subjects. *Diabetes*; 44:1126–1131.

Drucker DJ. (2003) Glucagon-like peptides: regulators of cell proliferation, differentiation, and apoptosis. *Mol Endocrinol*; 17:161–171.

Elrick H, Stimmler L, Hlad CJ Jr, Arai Y. (1964) Plasma insulin response to oral and intravenous glucose administration. *J Clin Endocrinol Metab*; 24:1076–1082.

Grossman S. (2009) Differentiating incretin therapies based on structure, activity, and metabolism: focus on liraglutide. *Pharmacotherapy*; 29 (12 Pt 2):25S–32S.

Nauck MA, Homberger E, Siegel EG, *et al.* (1986) Incretin effects of increasing glucose loads in man calculated from venous insulin and C-peptide responses. *J Clin Endocrinol Metab*; 63:492–498.

Vilsbøll T, Krarup T, Deacon CF, *et al.* (2001) Reduced postprandial concentrations of intact biologically active glucagon-like peptide 1 in type 2 diabetic patients. *Diabetes*; 50:609–613.

4 The Incretin Mimetics

The incretin-based therapies are unique among currently marketed drugs in combining a broad range of glucose-lowering effects without the limitations associated with some conventional therapies such as hypoglycaemia and weight gain.

Exenatide

Exenatide mechanism of action

The incretin mimetics lower blood glucose by mimicking the effects of the natural incretin hormone, glucagon-like peptide-1 (GLP-1). Exenatide was the first such agent to reach the market, launched in 2005 in the USA and 2007 in the UK. Exenatide is a synthetic form of exendin 4, a molecule that was originally isolated from Gila monster (*Heloderma suspectum*) venom. Exenatide is not an analogue of human GLP-1 sharing only 53% sequence identity (Figure 4.1), but the structural similarity is sufficient to allow it to bind to the GLP-1 receptor and mimic the broad range of glucoregulatory actions of GLP-1, while not acting as a substrate for dipeptidyl peptidase-4 (DPP-4).

Exenatide lowers fasting and postprandial glucose concentrations by a number of mechanisms, which it shares with GLP-1. In the pancreas, exenatide simultaneously stimulates insulin secretion from the beta cell and suppresses the hypersecretion of glucagon from the alpha cell, the latter reducing hepatic glucose production in the postprandial state. These actions only occur in the presence of elevated circulating glucose concentrations thereby minimizing the risk of hypoglycaemia. Like GLP-1, exenatide is associated with a slowing of gastric emptying and promotes a feeling of satiety, which can lead to weight loss in overweight individuals (Linnebjerg *et al.*, 2008). In animal studies, exenatide appears to promote pancreatic islet cell differentiation and inhibit beta-cell apoptosis, shifting the balance toward an increase in islet mass. As beta-cell mass cannot be measured non-invasively in humans, beta-cell function can only be determined from indirect measures such as the proinsulin:insulin ratio and the homeostasis model assessment of beta-cell function (HOMA-B). Although indirect, the consistency of the data from clinical

New Mechanisms in Glucose Control, First Edition. Anthony H. Barnett & Jenny Grice.
© 2011 Anthony H. Barnett & Jenny Grice. Published 2011 Blackwell Publishing Ltd.

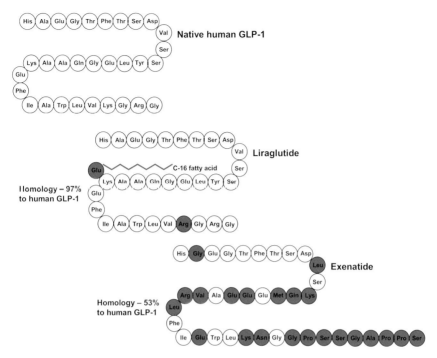

Figure 4.1 Structures of GLP-1 and the GLP-1 receptor agonists exenatide and liraglutide (shaded residues indicate differences from native GLP-1).

studies suggests that the GLP-1 receptor agonists as well as the DPP-4 inhibitors do improve beta-cell function (Drucker, 2006).

Exenatide clinical efficacy

The Phase 3 clinical efficacy studies that have been conducted with exenatide are listed in Table 4.1. Three 30-week, placebo-controlled studies evaluated exenatide (5 μg or 10 μg twice daily) as add-on therapy in overweight or obese patients not achieving adequate glycaemic control despite treatment with maximally effective doses of metformin (Defronzo *et al.*, 2005), a sulphonylurea (Buse *et al.*, 2004), or the combination of metformin and a sulphonylurea (Kendall *et al.*, 2005). After completion of the placebo-controlled phase, these studies continued into three long-term uncontrolled extension studies designed to demonstrate the durability of exenatide treatment (Blonde *et al.*, 2006; Buse *et al.*, 2007; Ratner *et al.*, 2006). In a placebo-controlled study of 16 weeks duration, exenatide was added to existing thiazolidinedione treatment, with or without metformin (Zinman *et al.*, 2007). In addition, three Phase 3, long-term active-comparator controlled studies have been conducted to establish the non-inferiority of exenatide treatment (10 μg twice daily) to insulin treatment (insulin glargine, once daily or biphasic insulin aspart, twice daily)

Table 4.1 Exenatide Phase 3 clinical efficacy studies

Reference	Duration (weeks)	n	Exenatide dose (bid)	Comparator agents	Baseline HbA$_{1c}$	Change in HbA$_{1c}$ (%)*	Change in body weight (Kg)*
Buse et al.	30	377	5 μg 10 μg	SU	8.6	−0.46 −0.86	−0.9 −1.6
DeFronzo et al.	30	336	5 μg 10 μg	Met	8.3	−0.40 −0.78	−1.6 −2.8
Kendall et al.	30	733	5 μg 10 μg	Met + SU	8.5	−0.55 −0.77	−1.6 −1.6
Zinman et al.	16	233	10 μg	TZD + Met	7.9	−0.89	−1.5
Heine et al.	26	549	10 μg	Met + SU (vs glargine)	8.2	−1.11	−2.3
Nauck et al.	52	501	10 μg	Met + SU (vs aspart)	8.6	−1.0	−5.4
Barnett et al.	16	138	10 μg	Met or SU (vs glargine)	8.95	−1.36	−2.2

*Changes in HbA$_{1c}$ (%) and body weight (Kg) are from baseline. Met, metformin; SU, sulphonylurea; TZD, thiazolidinedione

in patients with inadequate blood glucose control using oral agents (Barnett *et al.*, 2007; Heine *et al.*, 2005; Nauck *et al.*, 2006).

In the placebo-controlled trials, exenatide 10 μg was associated with reductions in HbA$_{1c}$ of 0.8−0.9% (Figure 4.2) demonstrating similar efficacy to currently available oral antidiabetes agents. All exenatide doses were associated with significant and sustained reductions in postprandial plasma glucose compared with placebo, and at the exenatide 10 μg dose, placebo-subtracted reductions in fasting plasma glucose were in the range of 1.0–1.4 mmol/L (Buse *et al.*, 2004; DeFronzo *et al.*, 2005; Kendall *et al.*, 2005). All the studies have also demonstrated improvements in surrogate measures of beta-cell function such as the proinsulin:insulin ratio and HOMA-B.

An important advantage of exenatide is that it is associated with weight loss and mean reductions of 1.5−2.8 kg were reported in the placebo-controlled trials (Figure 4.3). There was little or no increase in hypoglycaemia except as add-on to a sulphonylurea, and the antihyperglycaemic efficacy was sustained in open-label extension studies up to two years (Blonde *et al.*, 2006; Buse *et al.*, 2007; Ratner *et al.*, 2006). In addition, an improvement in low-density lipoprotein (LDL) and high-density lipoprotein (HDL) cholesterol, triglycerides and blood pressure was observed (Klonoff *et al.*, 2008). In the active-comparator studies, exenatide was able to achieve similar reductions in HbA$_{1c}$ to basal long-acting insulin and to biphasic insulin regimens and was associated with significant reductions in body weight. In the insulin glargine comparator trials, exenatide was associated with greater reductions in

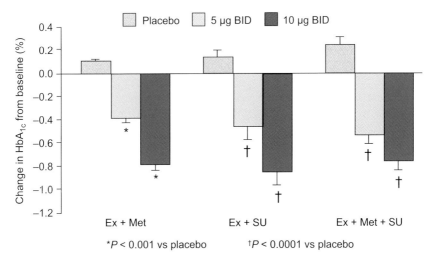

Figure 4.2 Exenatide effects on glycaemic control in combination with oral antidiabetes agents (Buse *et al.*, 2004; DeFronzo *et al.*, 2005; Kendall *et al.*, 2005).

postprandial plasma glucose excursions, whereas insulin glargine was associated with greater reductions in levels of fasting plasma glucose (Barnett *et al.*, 2007; Heine *et al.*, 2005).

A long-acting release formulation of exenatide is also in development, which encapsulates exenatide in polymer microspheres that gradually disintegrate in the body to release exenatide. This formulation is suitable for once-weekly subcutaneous injection and results in significantly greater improvements in glycaemic control than exenatide given twice a day, with no

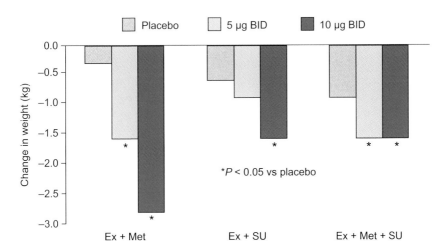

Figure 4.3 Exenatide reductions in body weight in combination with oral antidiabetes agents (Buse *et al.*, 2004; DeFronzo *et al.*, 2005; Kendall *et al.*, 2005).

increased risk of hypoglycaemia and with similar reductions in body weight (Drucker *et al.*, 2008; Kim *et al.*, 2007). Exenatide once weekly is also associated with less nausea, probably because of more stable circulating levels of exenatide. However, due to a larger 23 gauge needle (compared with 31 gauge needle for injection of immediate release exenatide) injection site bruising can occur more frequently. An open-label, randomized trial comparing once-weekly exenatide with insulin glargine in people with type 2 diabetes has been completed. The results suggest that weekly exenatide may be a suitable alternative to insulin in patients inadequately controlled on existing treatment, particularly where weight loss is desirable (Diamant *et al.*, 2010). In a further Phase 3 study, once-weekly exenatide also provided greater HbA$_{1c}$ reductions compared with maximum dose oral sitagliptin or pioglitazone in patients inadequately controlled on metformin monotherapy (Bergenstal *et al.*, 2010). However, in both trials more patients discontinued exenatide than the comparator therapy due to adverse effects.

Exenatide safety and tolerability

Nausea is the most common tolerability issue associated with exenatide, reported by at least one third of patients, and is thought to be associated with the delayed gastric emptying. It is usually mild and can be minimized by starting with the 5 µg dose for the first month before titrating up to the 10 µg dose (Fineman *et al.*, 2004). As both exenatide and sulphonylureas stimulate the beta cells to produce more insulin, hypoglycaemia can be a problem when these agents are used in combination. Slow titration can help to reduce hypoglycaemic episodes, and the risk can also be reduced by lowering the dose of the sulphonylurea. There have been rare reports of acute pancreatitis during use of exenatide (MHRA, 2008) and as is true with all new drugs, careful attention to clinical effects that emerge over time will be necessary to ensure the drug's safety.

Exenatide advantages and disadvantages

The major disadvantage of exenatide is that it is injected twice daily and must be administered 30 to 60 minutes before the first and last meals of the day. Exenatide raises insulin levels rapidly (within 10 minutes of administration) with levels subsiding substantially over the next 2 hours. As a dose taken after meals has a much smaller effect on blood sugar than one taken beforehand, exenatide should not be used after eating a meal. Delayed gastric emptying with exenatide may also result in a reduction in the rate and extent of absorption of orally administered drugs. Mild to moderate nausea is common with the initiation of exenatide therapy, but tends to diminish with continued exposure. Besides this, exenatide does have a number of advantages that make it more convenient than insulin. First, the volumes administered are small and injection site pain is uncommon. Second, there is no need for bottles and syringes; exenatide is supplied as a pre-filled pen device. Third, unlike insulin there is no need for dose adjustments in response to the size of meals or activity.

The major advantage of exenatide is that it is the first glucose-lowering agent to demonstrate substantial and sustained weight loss. Compared with the sulphonylureas and insulin, exenatide is not associated with hypoglycaemia as an adverse effect. Based on data from animal studies there is also a possibility that exenatide therapy may be able to preserve or even restore beta-cell function.

Exenatide current indications

Exenatide is indicated for the treatment of type 2 diabetes in combination with metformin and/or sulphonylureas in patients who have not achieved adequate glycaemic control on maximally tolerated doses of these oral therapies (Byetta SmPC, 2009). In the most recent guidance from the National Institute for Health and Clinical Excellence (NICE), exenatide is an alternative to insulin or other third-line therapy in obese patients (body mass index (BMI) of at least 35 kg/m^2) who have failed to achieve adequate glycaemic control on maximal dose oral antidiabetes agents (NICE, 2009). It may also be considered in a patient with a BMI less than 35 kg/m^2 if weight loss would benefit other comorbidities, or insulin therapy is not appropriate or acceptable (NICE, 2009).

Liraglutide

Liraglutide mechanism of action

Liraglutide is an analogue of human GLP-1 created by substituting one amino acid and adding a fatty acid side chain (Figure 4.1). The resultant molecule has 97% sequence identity with human GLP-1. The fatty acid side chain increases non-covalent binding to albumin after injection, which protects liraglutide from degradation by DPP-4 as well as reducing clearance. The structural modifications also allow liraglutide to self-associate into heptamers, which results in slow absorption from the subcutaneous injection site. These three characteristics combine to give the compound a plasma half-life of 10–12 hours in humans, compared with approximately 2 minutes for native GLP-1 and 2.4 hours for exenatide. The prolonged action makes liraglutide suitable for once-daily dosing. Liraglutide retains affinity for the GLP-1 receptor and produces the effects expected of a GLP-1 agonist in patients with type 2 diabetes including improved glycaemic control, increased meal-related and glucose-stimulated insulin secretion, suppression of glucagon, weight loss, delayed gastric emptying and appetite suppression, and enhanced beta-cell function (for a review, see Rossi and Nicolucci, 2009). Due to the high degree of homology between liraglutide and native GLP-1, the risk of antibody formation is lower than with exenatide (Marre *et al.*, 2009; Russell-Jones *et al.*, 2009); however, the clinical relevance of antibodies to either agent is not yet known.

Liraglutide clinical efficacy

The clinical efficacy of liraglutide has been evaluated in the Liraglutide Effect and Action in Diabetes (LEAD) programme. This was designed to assess the efficacy and safety of liraglutide across the continuum of type 2 diabetes care,

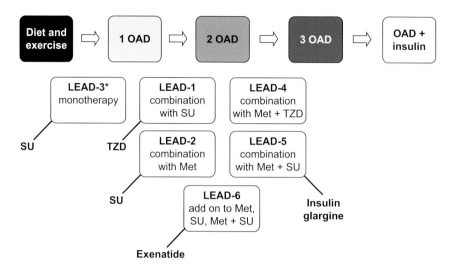

Figure 4.4 Liraglutide Effect and Action in Diabetes (LEAD) Phase 3 programme. Met, metformin. OAD, oral antidiabetes agent. SU, sulphonylurea. TZD, thiazolidinedione. *Liraglutide is not licensed for use as monotherapy.

both as monotherapy (off license) and in combination with commonly used oral antidiabetes agents, in a series of five randomized, double-blind, controlled trials and one open-label trial in more than 6800 people, 4600 of whom received liraglutide treatment (Figure 4.4). A unique feature of the LEAD programme was that as well as a placebo arm, all of the studies except one had active comparators.

All the LEAD trials have demonstrated HbA_{1c} reductions greater than 1% with the therapeutic dose of liraglutide in patients with baseline HbA_{1c} levels in the low to mid 8% range (Figure 4.5). In LEAD 1, liraglutide was added to a sulphonylurea and the active comparator was rosiglitazone (Marre *et al.*, 2009). Liraglutide at doses of 1.2 or 1.8 mg/day achieved a statistically significant twofold greater reduction in HbA_{1c} than rosiglitazone. In LEAD 2, liraglutide was added to metformin with glimepiride as the active comparator (Nauck *et al.*, 2009). Equivalent reductions in HbA_{1c} were observed between the 1.8 mg liraglutide dose and the sulphonylurea. LEAD 3 was the only liraglutide monotherapy trial and compared liraglutide 1.2 mg and 1.8 mg with glimepiride for 52 weeks (Garber *et al.*, 2009). (Liraglutide is not currently licensed for use as monotherapy.) Liraglutide 1.8 mg reduced HbA_{1c} by approximately 1.1%, a twofold greater reduction than glimepiride. Liraglutide 1.2 mg was associated with a reduction in HbA1c of 0.8%. However, it should be remembered that patients were not necessarily drug-naïve when they were switched to glimepiride monotherapy at study entry, which may account for the less than expected efficacy with glimepiride. The LEAD 4 trial evaluated liraglutide in patients treated with rosiglitazone and metformin and was the only trial without an active comparator (Zinman *et al.*, 2009). Both liraglutide

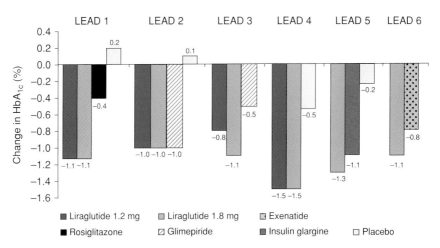

Figure 4.5 Change in HbA$_{1c}$ with liraglutide 1.2 mg and 1.8 mg in the LEAD trials.

1.2 mg and 1.8 mg achieved significantly greater reductions in HbA$_{1c}$ compared with placebo plus dual oral agent therapy in the order of approximately 1.5%. In all the above trials, a similar pattern was observed for the effects of liraglutide on fasting plasma glucose levels, with significant benefits for liraglutide versus the active comparator, particularly in comparison with a sulphonlyurea (Nauck *et al.*, 2009).

The LEAD 5 trial was an open-label trial, which compared liraglutide 1.8 mg with insulin glargine in patients receiving dual oral agent therapy with metformin and a sulphonylurea (Russell-Jones *et al.*, 2009). Although insulin glargine achieved greater reductions in fasting plasma glucose, liraglutide was associated with significantly greater reductions in HbA$_{1c}$ as a result of its combined effects on fasting and postprandial plasma glucose.

The final trial was LEAD 6, which was a head-to-head comparison of subcutaneous liraglutide 1.8 mg once a day with exenatide 10 µg twice a day (Buse *et al.*, 2009). Liraglutide was associated with a significantly greater reduction in HbA$_{1c}$ compared with exenatide (1.12% vs 0.79%, respectively). Significantly greater reductions in fasting plasma glucose were also achieved reflecting liraglutide's action as a 24-hour GLP-1 receptor agonist. Exenatide achieved greater reductions in postprandial plasma glucose as a result of its more rapid time–action profile.

Weight reductions across the LEAD 1 to 4 trials were in the order of 2–3 kg with liraglutide compared with increases of 0.6–2.6 kg for the active comparators. The only trial that did not display a reduction in weight was LEAD 1 in which liraglutide plus glimepiride treatment was weight neutral (Marre *et al.*, 2009). In LEAD 5, liraglutide was associated with a significant reduction in body weight compared with insulin, and in LEAD 6, both liraglutide and exenatide achieved similar reductions in body weight of approximately 3 kg at the end of the 26-week trial. Improvements in parameters assessing beta-cell

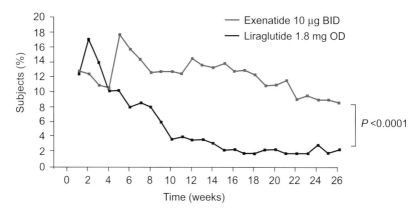

Figure 4.6 Nausea associated with liraglutide is transient compared with exenatide (Buse *et al.*, 2009). Data are number (%) of patients exposed to treatment (safety population). Reproduced from Buse *et al.* (2009) with permission from Elsevier.

function were consistently shown with liraglutide treatment across all trials. Furthermore, reductions in systolic blood pressure were reported.

Liraglutide safety and tolerability

Across the LEAD trials, nausea was the most commonly reported adverse event, but was usually mild to moderate and only led to the withdrawal of 2.8% of patients. The head-to-head comparison with exenatide suggests that the incidence may be lower with liraglutide (Buse *et al.*, 2009). In the early weeks of the study, both exenatide and liraglutide were associated with rates of nausea of 15–18% with peaks occurring during periods of drug titration (Figure 4.6). Liraglutide then demonstrated a progressive decline in nausea rate to 2% which was maintained for the duration of the trial. In comparison, rates of nausea with exenatide only declined to 8–10%. It has been suggested that the lower rate of nausea with liraglutide is probably related to its more stable and longer acting GLP-1 activity. A few cases (less than 0.2%) of acute pancreatitis have been reported during long-term clinical trials with liraglutide and at this time a causal relationship between liraglutide and pancreatitis can neither be established nor excluded.

Liraglutide advantages and disadvantages

The disadvantages of liraglutide for the most part mirror those of exenatide and include the injection formulation, frequency of gastrointestinal adverse events, and the lack of extensive clinical data, although the latter is being addressed in the ongoing Liraglutide Effect and Action in Diabetes: Evaluation of Cardiovascular Outcome Results (LEADER) trial. Liraglutide also shares the advantages of exenatide including glucose-lowering efficacy in combination with weight loss and a negligible incidence of hypoglycaemia unless used in combination with a sulphonylurea. The advantages of liraglutide over exenatide are that injection is only once daily and a lower rate of nausea. In

addition, administration is not restricted to a meal time; the patient can se-
lect the most suitable injection time and then continue to inject at that time
each day. Finally, the marketing authorization for liraglutide covers a wider
indication than exenatide, which may only be used with metformin and/or a
sulphonylurea or thiazolidinedione.

Liraglutide current indications

Liraglutide was licensed in the European Union in 2009 and is available as a
pre-filled pen. It is indicated for the treatment of adults with type 2 diabetes
in combination with metformin or a sulphonylurea in patients with insufficient glycaemic control despite maximal tolerated dose monotherapy, and in
combination with metformin and a sulphonylurea or metformin and a thiazolidinedione in patients with insufficient glycaemic control despite dual therapy (Victoza SmPC, 2010). To improve gastrointestinal tolerability, the starting
dose is 0.6 mg liraglutide daily, which is increased to 1.2 mg daily after at least
one week. Some patients may benefit from an increase in dose from 1.2 mg to
1.8 mg daily. Although liraglutide was not licensed in time for inclusion in the
NICE update to its clinical guideline on the management of type 2 diabetes, in
October 2010 NICE released a single technology appraisal in which liraglutide
1.2 mg daily in triple therapy regimens (in combination with metformin and a
sulphonylurea, or metformin and a thiazolidinedione) was recommended as
a treatment option in people with type 2 diabetes if they have an HbA_{1c} of at
least 7.5% and a BMI of 35 kg/m^2 or more (NICE TAG 203, 2010).The drug
may also be used in individuals with a BMI below 35 kg/m^2 if therapy with
insulin would have significant occupational implications, or to achieve levels
of weight loss beneficial in treating other obesity-related comorbidities.

In addition, NICE recommended that liraglutide could be used second line
where metformin or sulphonylurea is contraindicated or not tolerated and
where both a thiazolidinedione and a DPP-4 inhibitor are contraindicated or
not tolerated. Whilst seemingly very restrictive this appears to allow for situ-
ations where weight gain must be avoided at all costs (e.g. in cases of severe
chronic obstructive sleep apnoea) and in which thiazolidinediones, sulphonylureas and insulin would therefore not be advisable. If significant clinical benefit would be expected from weight loss in the author's opinion this
would allow for a metformin/liraglutide second-line combination in these
types of cases.

In 2009, the Scottish Medicines Consortium completed its assessment of the
product, recommending liraglutide for restricted use as a third-line antidiabetes agent (SMC, 2009).

Place in therapy of the incretin mimetics

The incretin mimetics offer an alternative approach for patients with type 2
diabetes not adequately controlled with diet plus metformin and/or a sulphonylurea. Of particular importance for patients is the finding that incretin-
based therapies depend absolutely on glucose for their actions, a major

distinction between them and other insulin secretagogues such as sulphony-lureas. This glucose dependency provides a low risk for hypoglycaemia. Exe-natide and liraglutide are also able to promote satiety so that the patient eats less, and to slow gastric emptying so that less glucose reaches the intestine and bloodstream after a meal. Theoretically, exenatide and liraglutide may be useful in slowing the progression of type 2 diabetes due to their apparent ben-eficial effects on beta-cell function. However, until this has been confirmed in long-term clinical trials the target population for these agents is likely to be patients poorly controlled with diet plus metformin and/or a sulphonylurea or thiazolidinedione who are reluctant to move to insulin therapy out of fear of hypoglycaemia, weight gain and/or frequent glucose monitoring.

References

Barnett AH, Burger J, Johns D, *et al.* (2007) Tolerability and efficacy of exenatide and titrated insulin glargine in adult patients with type 2 diabetes previously uncontrolled with metformin or a sulfonylurea: a multinational, randomized, open-label, two-period, crossover noninferiority trial. *Clin Ther*; 29:2333–2348.

Bergenstal RM, Wysham C, Macconell L, *et al.* (2010) Efficacy and safety of exenatide once weekly versus sitagliptin or pioglitazone as an adjunct to metformin for treatment of type 2 diabetes (DURATION-2): a randomised trial. *Lancet*; 376:431–439.

Blonde L, Klein EJ, Han J, *et al.* (2006) Interim analysis of the effects of exenatide treatment on A1c, weight and cardiovascular risk factors over 82 weeks in 314 overweight patients with type 2 diabetes. *Diabetes Obes Metab*; 8:436–447.

Buse JB, Henry RR, Han J, *et al.* (2004) Effect of exenatide (exendin-4) on glycemic con-trol over 30 weeks in sulfonylurea-treated patients with type 2 diabetes. *Diabetes Care*; 27:2628–2635.

Buse JB, Klonoff DC, Nielsen LL, *et al.* (2007) Metabolic effects of two years of exenatide treatment on diabetes, obesity and hepatic biomarkers in patients with type 2 diabetes: an interim analysis of data from the open-label, uncontrolled extension of three double-blind, placebo-controlled trials. *Clin Ther*; 29:139–153.

Buse JB, Rosenstock J, Sesti G, *et al.*; LEAD-6 Study Group. (2009) Liraglutide once a day versus exenatide twice a day for type 2 diabetes: a 26-week randomised, parallel-group, multinational, open-label trial (LEAD-6). *Lancet*; 374:39–47.

Byetta SmPC (2009) Eli Lilly and Company Limited. Byetta 5 micrograms solution for injection, prefilled pen. Byetta 10 micrograms solution for injection, prefilled pen. Summary of Product Characteristics (UK). Available at: http://emc.medicines.org.uk/medicine/19257#PRODUCTINFO

DeFronzo RA, Ratner RE, Han J, *et al.* (2005) Effects of exenatide (exendin-4) on glycemic control and weight over 30 weeks in metformin-treated patients with type 2 diabetes. *Diabetes Care*; 28:1092–1100.

Diamant M, Van Gaal L, Stranks S, *et al.* (2010) Once weekly exenatide compared with insulin glargine titrated to target in patients with type 2 diabetes (DURATION-3): an open-label randomised trial. *Lancet*; 375:2234–2243.

Drucker DJ. (2006) The biology of incretin hormones. *Cell Metab;* 3:153–165.

Drucker DJ, Buse JB, Taylor K, *et al.*; DURATION-1 Study Group. (2008) Exenatide once weekly versus twice daily for the treatment of type 2 diabetes: a randomised, open-label, non-inferiority study. *Lancet*; 372:1240–1250.

Fineman MS, Shen LZ, Taylor K, *et al.* (2004) Effectiveness of progressive dose-escalation of exenatide (exendin-4) in reducing dose-limiting side effects in subjects with type 2 diabetes. *Diabetes Metab Res Rev*; 20:411–417.

Garber A, Henry R, Ratner R, *et al.*; LEAD-3 (Mono) Study Group (2009) Liraglutide versus glimepiride monotherapy for type 2 diabetes (LEAD-3 Mono): a randomised, 52-week, phase III, double-blind, parallel-treatment trial. *Lancet*; 373:473–481.

Heine RJ, Van Gaal LF, Johns D, *et al.*; GWAA Study Group (2005) Exenatide versus insulin glargine in patients with suboptimally controlled type 2 diabetes: a randomized trial. *Ann Intern Med*; 143:559–569.

Kendall DM, Riddle MC, Rosenstock J, *et al.* (2005) Effects of exenatide (exendin-4) on glycemic control over 30 weeks in patients with type 2 diabetes treated with metformin and a sulfonylurea. *Diabetes Care*; 28:1083–1091.

Kim D, Macconell L, Zhuang D, *et al.* (2007) Effect of once-weekly dosing of a long-acting release formulation of exenatide on glucose control and body weight in subjects with type 2 diabetes. *Diabetes Care*; 30:1487–1493.

Klonoff DC, Buse JB, Nielsen LL, *et al.* (2008) Exenatide effects on diabetes, obesity, cardio-vascular risk factors and hepatic biomarkers in patients with type 2 diabetes treated for at least 3 years. *Curr Med Res Opin*; 24:275–286.

Linnebjerg H, Park S, Kothare PA, *et al.* (2008) Effect of exenatide on gastric emptying and relationship to postprandial glycemia in type 2 diabetes. *Regul Pept*; 151:123–129.

Marre M, Shaw J, Brändle M, *et al.*; LEAD-1 SU Study Group (2009) Liraglutide, a once-daily human GLP-1 analogue, added to a sulphonylurea over 26 weeks produces greater improvements in glycaemic and weight control compared with adding rosiglitazone or placebo in subjects with type 2 diabetes (LEAD-1 SU). *Diabetic Med*; 26:268–278.

Medicines and Healthcare products Regulatory Agency (MHRA) (2008) Exenatide (Byetta): risk of acute pancreatitis. Drug Safety Update 2008; 1:5. Available from: http://cks.library.nhs.uk/media/drug_safety_update/110.pdf. Last accessed February 2010.

National Institute for Health and Clinical Excellence (NICE) (2009) Type 2 diabetes: newer agents for blood glucose control. NICE short clinical guidelines 87. Available from: http://www.nice.org.uk/nicemedia/pdf/CG87NICEGuideline.pdf. Last accessed February 2010.

National Institute for Health and Clinical Excellence (NICE) (2010) Liraglutide for the treatment of type 2 diabetes mellitus. NICE technology appraisal guidance 203. Available from: http://www.nice.org.uk/nicemedia/live/13248/51259/51259.pdf. Last accessed December 2010.

Nauck MA, Duraan S, Kim D, *et al.* (2006) A comparison of twice-daily exenatide and biphasic insulin aspart in patients with type 2 diabetes who were suboptimally controlled with sulfonylurea and metformin: a non-inferiority study. *Diabetologia*; 50:259–267.

Nauck M, Frid A, Hermansen K, *et al.*; LEAD-2 Study Group (2009) Efficacy and safety comparison of liraglutide, glimepiride, and placebo, all in combination with metformin in type 2 diabetes mellitus (LEAD-2 Met). *Diabetes Care*; 32:84–90.

Ratner RE, Maggs D, Nielsen LL, *et al.* (2006) Long-term effects of exenatide therapy over 82 weeks on glycaemic control and weight in over-weight metformin-treated patients with type 2 diabetes mellitus. *Diabetes Obes Metab*; 8:419–428.

Rossi MC, Nicolucci A. (2009) Liraglutide in type 2 diabetes: from pharmacological development to clinical practice. *Acta Biomed*; 80:93–101.

Russell-Jones D, Vaag A, Schmitz O, *et al.*; Liraglutide Effect and Action in Diabetes 5 (LEAD-5) met+SU Study Group (2009) Liraglutide vs insulin glargine and placebo in combination with metformin and sulphonylurea therapy in type 2 diabetes mellitus: a randomised controlled trial (LEAD-5 met+SU). *Diabetologia*; 52:2046–2055.

Scottish Medicines Consortium (SMC) (2009). Liraglutide 6mg/mL prefilled pen for injection (3mL) (Victoza®). December 2009. Available from: http://www.scottishmedicines.org.uk/files/liraglutideVictozaFINALNovember2009revised011209.pdf

Victoza SmPC (2010) Novo Nordisk Limited. Victoza 6 mg/ml solution for injection in pre-filled pen. Summary of Product Characteristics (UK). Available at: http://emc.medicines.org.uk/medicine/21986/SPC/#INDICATIONS

Zinman B, Hoogwerf BJ, Garcia SD, *et al.* (2007) The effect of adding exenatide to a thiazolidinedione in suboptimally controlled type 2 diabetes: a randomized trial. *Ann Intern Med*; 146:477–485.

Zinman B, Gerich J, Buse JB, *et al.*; LEAD-4 Study Investigators (2009) Efficacy and safety of the human GLP-1 analog liraglutide in combination with metformin and TZD in patients with type 2 diabetes mellitus (LEAD-4 Met+TZD). *Diabetes Care*; 32:1224–1230.

5 Dipeptidyl Peptidase-4 Inhibitors

Mechanism of action

The dipeptidyl peptidase-4 (DPP-4) inhibitors also known as incretin enhancers, increase active levels of the incretin hormones glucagon-like peptide-1 (GLP-1) and gastric inhibitory peptide (GIP) by inhibiting the enzyme responsible for their breakdown. The net result is higher levels of endogenous GLP-1 with a longer half-life. In Europe, sitagliptin and vildagliptin were the first two agents in this class to be approved in 2007 and 2008, respectively. Saxagliptin approval followed in July 2009, and alogliptin was approved in Japan in April 2010. Linagliptin has completed pivotal Phase 3 trials and a number of other DPP-4 inhibitors are in various stages of development.

The mode of action is a competitive, reversible inhibition of DPP-4 providing up to 90% inhibition of plasma DPP-4 activity during a 24-hour period (Deacon and Holst, 2006). Although they target the same biochemical pathway as the incretin mimetics, the DPP-4 inhibitors display some differences, which are thought to be explained by the fact that the DPP-4 inhibitors raise GLP-1 levels to physiological levels, whereas the incretin mimetics can achieve levels at least fivefold higher. Glucoregulatory actions of the DPP-4 inhibitors include stimulation of insulin secretion, inhibition of glucagon secretion, and improvement in beta-cell function based on surrogate markers (Table 5.1). In contrast to the incretin mimetics, DPP-4 inhibitors do not appear to mediate all the glucoregulatory actions of native GLP-1, having little or no effect on gastric emptying or satiety. This is thought to partly explain their weight neutrality in the clinical setting.

The DPP-4 inhibitors can be divided into two classes based on the presence or absence of a cyanopyrrolidine ring, which results in some differences in their actions. Vildagliptin and saxagliptin possess a cyanopyrrolidine group, whereas sitagliptin, alogliptin and linagliptin do not. The latter are highly selective for DPP-4, whereas the selectivity of saxagliptin and vildagliptin is somewhat less, although this is not thought to be clinically relevant. Another difference between the two groups of DPP-4 inhibitors relates to their method of elimination. Sitagliptin and alogliptin are excreted by the kidneys, mostly as unchanged molecules. In contrast, saxagliptin and vildagliptin are

New Mechanisms in Glucose Control, First Edition. Anthony H. Barnett & Jenny Grice.
© 2011 Anthony H. Barnett & Jenny Grice. Published 2011 Blackwell Publishing Ltd.

Table 5.1 Comparison of the properties of the incretin mimetics and DPP-4 inhibitors in patients with type 2 diabetes

Action	Incretin mimetics	DPP-4 inhibitors
Route of administration	Subcutaneous injection	Oral
Duration of GLP-1 elevation	Up to 24 hours	3–6 hours postprandial
GLP-1 concentration	Supraphysiological ($>$ 5)	Close to physiological
Insulin secretion	Enhanced	Enhanced
Glucagon secretion	Suppressed	Suppressed
Postprandial hyperglycaemia	Reduced	Reduced
Gastric emptying	Slowed significantly	No effect
Appetite	Suppressed	No effect
Satiety	Induced	No effect
HbA$_{1c}$ reduction	0.8–1.5%	0.5–0.8%
Body weight	Reduced	No effect
Beta-cell function	Preservation*; proinsulin:insulin ratio improved clinically	Preservation*; proinsulin:insulin ratio improved clinically
Gastrointestinal side-effects	Frequent	Rare

*Demonstrated in animal models

metabolized. Saxagliptin has an active metabolite, which is metabolized in the liver and kidney, while the vildagliptin metabolite is inactive and mostly excreted by the kidney. Linagliptin is unique among the DPP-4 inhibitors in having a primarily non-renal route of excretion. This may make it particularly suitable for use in patients with significant renal impairment.

DPP-4 inhibitor clinical efficacy

Sitagliptin

The pivotal sitagliptin clinical efficacy trials for European registration comprised two monotherapy studies (Aschner *et al.*, 2006; Raz *et al.*, 2006), two placebo-controlled combination studies (Charbonnel *et al.*, 2006; Rosenstock *et al.*, 2006), and one active-controlled combination study (Nauck *et al.*, 2007). The two monotherapy trials had durations of 18 and 24 weeks and compared sitagliptin 100 mg or 200 mg once daily with placebo (Aschner *et al.*, 2006; Raz *et al.*, 2006). Sitagliptin significantly reduced HbA$_{1c}$ by 0.5–0.9% compared with placebo, with few adverse events, no weight gain, and no significant increase in hypoglycaemia.

In two combination studies, sitagliptin was added to metformin (Charbonnel *et al.*, 2006) or pioglitazone (Rosenstock *et al.*, 2006) and compared to the effect of addition of placebo. These studies had 24-week durations, with an extension to 104 weeks in the metformin combination study. Mean

Table 5.2 HbA$_{1c}$-lowering efficacy of sitagliptin in combination with other antidiabetes agents

Sitagliptin trial	Treatments	Duration (weeks)	Baseline HbA$_{1c}$ (%)	Mean change from baseline HbA$_{1c}$ (%)	Mean difference from comparator (%)
Charbonnel et al., 2006	Sitagliptin 100 mg + metformin	24	8.0	−0.67	−0.65
	Placebo + metformin		8.0	−0.02	
Rosenstock et al., 2006	Sitagliptin 100 mg + pioglitazone	24	8.1	−0.85	−0.70
	Placebo + pioglitazone		8.0	−0.15	
Nauck et al., 2007	Sitagliptin 100 mg + metformin	52	7.5	−0.67	–
	Glipizide + metformin		7.5	−0.67	

placebo-subtracted reductions in HbA$_{1c}$ with sitagliptin were 0.65% (Charbonnel *et al.*, 2006) and 0.70% (Rosenstock *et al.*, 2006) (Table 5.2) with no increased rates of hypoglycaemia or weight gain. Sitagliptin has also been shown to be effective when combined with metformin as initial therapy for type 2 diabetes (Goldstein *et al.*, 2007).

In a 52-week active-comparator study, patients not achieving adequate glycaemic control on a metformin dose of at least 1500 mg/day were randomized to sitagliptin 100 mg once daily or glipizide, which was initiated at a dose of 5 mg/day. Up-titration of glipizide was performed over 18 weeks to a maximum dose of 20 mg, after which no increase in glipizide dose was permitted. Sitagliptin added to ongoing metformin therapy demonstrated an identical 0.67% HbA$_{1c}$ reduction to glipizide plus metformin therapy in a patient population with predominantly mild to moderate hyperglycaemia (Nauck *et al.*, 2007). In this study, 187 (32.0%) glipizide-treated patients reported 657 episodes of hypoglycaemia compared with 29 (4.9%) sitagliptin-treated patients who reported 50 episodes of hypoglycaemia. At 52 weeks, body weight was significantly reduced with sitagliptin (-1.5 kg) and significantly increased with glipizide (+1.1 kg) relative to baseline (Figure 5.1).

In all the pivotal sitagliptin studies, greater reductions in HbA$_{1c}$ were achieved in patients with higher HbA$_{1c}$ levels at baseline (Figure 5.2). Sitagliptin therapy reduced both fasting and postprandial plasma glucose, in association with improvements in the proinsulin:insulin ratio and homeostatic model assessment of beta-cell function (HOMA-B).

Vildagliptin

In an extensive clinical trial programme, vildagliptin at 50 mg once or twice daily and 100 mg once daily has been assessed in a number of

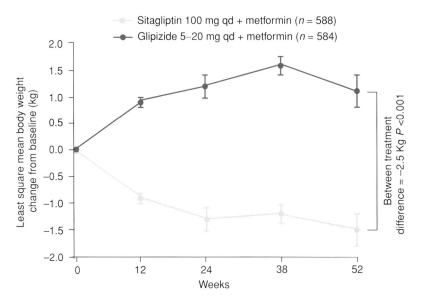

Figure 5.1 Effects of sitagliptin versus glipizide on body weight in patients with type 2 diabetes. Reproduced from Nauck *et al*. (2007) with permission from Wiley-Blackwell.

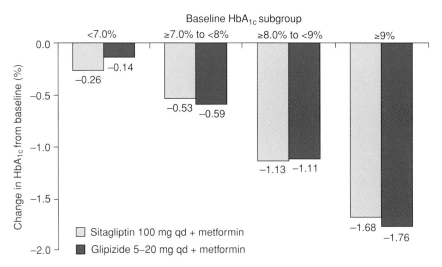

Figure 5.2 Mean HbA$_{1c}$ change ($\pm$ SE) from baseline at Week 52 by baseline HbA$_{1c}$ subgroups in the sitagliptin active-comparator study with glipizide. Reproduced from Nauck *et al*. (2007) with permission from Wiley-Blackwell.

placebo-controlled and active-comparator monotherapy studies (Dejager *et al.*, 2007; Pi-Sunyer *et al.*, 2007; Rosenstock *et al.*, 2007a; Schweizer *et al.*, 2007). Pooled data from these monotherapy trials in 1469 drug-naïve patients showed that vildagliptin 100 mg daily produced an adjusted mean change in HbA_{1c} of -1.0% at 24 weeks from a mean baseline value of 8.6% (Rosenstock and Fitchet, 2008). Two active-controlled monotherapy studies have compared vildagliptin 50 mg twice daily with either metformin 1000 mg twice daily (Schweizer *et al.*, 2007) or rosiglitazone 8 mg once daily (Rosenstock *et al.*, 2007a). Vildagliptin did not demonstrate non-inferiority to metformin in the one-year trial, although significant reductions in HbA_{1c} from baseline were achieved (Schweizer *et al.*, 2007). In contrast, in a 24-week study, vildagliptin was as effective as rosiglitazone with adjusted mean changes in HbA_{1c} of -1.1% versus -1.3% from a mean baseline of 8.7% (Rosenstock *et al.*, 2007a).

In a series of 24-week, 3-arm studies, vildagliptin 50 mg once daily, vildagliptin 50 mg twice daily and placebo have been compared as add-on combination therapy in patients with inadequate glycaemic control on metformin (Bosi *et al.*, 2007), a sulphonylurea (Garber *et al.*, 2008), or a thiazolidinedione (Garber *et al.*, 2007) (Table 5.3). In patients on metformin monotherapy, the two vildagliptin doses significantly decreased HbA_{1c} relative to placebo by 0.7% and 1.1%, respectively, although the difference between doses was not statistically significant (Bosi *et al.*, 2007). As add-on to glimepiride 4 mg per day, both vildagliptin doses in combination produced reductions in HbA_{1c} of 0.6% at 24 weeks, which were statistically significant compared with the 0.1% HbA_{1c} increase in the glimepiride plus placebo group (Garber *et al.*, 2008). Added to a maximum dose of pioglitazone, vildagliptin doses produced significant reductions from baseline of 0.8% and 1.0%, respectively, compared with a 0.3% reduction in patients receiving placebo plus pioglitazone (Garber *et al.*, 2007).

In a study of vildagliptin 50 mg twice daily or placebo as add-on to insulin, HbA_{1c} was reduced by 0.5% with vildagliptin at 24 weeks compared with 0.2% for placebo (Fonseca *et al.*, 2007). The improvements in HbA_{1c} with vildagliptin occurred in association with a lower total daily insulin dose and no episodes of significant hypoglycaemia compared with six episodes in those treated with insulin plus placebo.

A 24-week study has evaluated vildagliptin and pioglitazone as dual therapy compared with either agent as monotherapy in drug-naïve patients with type 2 diabetes (Rosenstock *et al.*, 2007b). From baseline to 24 weeks the vildagliptin 100 mg/day monotherapy group demonstrated a statistically significant reduction in HbA_{1c} of 1.1% compared with 1.4% for pioglitazone 30 mg/day monotherapy. Dual therapy demonstrated a 1.9% reduction in HbA_{1c} for the high dose dual therapy group (vildagliptin 100 mg plus pioglitazone 30 mg daily) and 1.7% in the low dose dual therapy group (vildagliptin 50 mg plus pioglitazone 15 mg daily).

Two active-comparator trials in patients with inadequate glycaemic control while receiving a stable metformin dose (at least 1500 mg/day) have

Table 5.3 HbA$_{1c}$-lowering efficacy of vildagliptin in combination with other antidiabetes agents

Vildagliptin trial	Treatments	Duration (weeks)	Baseline HbA$_{1c}$ (%)	Mean change from baseline HbA$_{1c}$ (%)	Mean difference from comparator (%)
Bosi et al., 2007	Vildagliptin 50 mg + metformin	24	8.4	−0.5	−0.7
	Vildagliptin 100 mg + metformin		8.4	−0.9	−1.1
	Placebo + metformin		8.3	0.2	
Garber et al., 2008	Vildagliptin 50 mg + glimepiride	24	8.6	−0.58	−0.64
	Vildagliptin 100 mg + glimepiride		8.6	−0.63	−0.70
	Placebo + glimepiride		8.5	0.07	
Garber et al., 2007	Vildagliptin 50 mg + pioglitazone	24	8.6	−0.76	−0.46
	Vildagliptin 100 mg + pioglitazone		8.7	−0.97	−0.67
	Placebo + pioglitazone		8.7	−0.30	
Fonseca et al., 2007	Vildagliptin 100 mg + insulin	24	8.5	−0.51	−0.27
	Placebo + insulin		8.5	−0.24	
Rosenstock et al., 2007	Vildagliptin 50 mg + pioglitazone 15 mg	24	8.76	−1.67	−0.26
	Vildagliptin 100 mg + pioglitazone 30 mg		8.77	−1.93	−0.55
	Vildagliptin 100 mg + placebo		8.6	−1.08	
	Pioglitazone 30 mg + placebo		8.69	−1.39	
Bolli et al., 2008	Vildagliptin 100 mg + metformin	24	8.4	−0.88	0.10
	Pioglitazone 30 mg + metformin		8.4	−0.98	
Ferrannini et al., 2009	Vildagliptin 100 mg + metformin	52	7.3	−0.44	
	Glimepiride + metformin		7.3	−0.53	

evaluated vildagliptin compared with pioglitazone (Bolli et al., 2008) and compared with glimepiride (Ferrannini et al., 2009). In the 24-week pioglitazone active comparator study, non-inferiority of vildagliptin to pioglitazone as add-on to metformin was established (Bolli et al., 2008). In a large two-year study, a pre-planned interim analysis at one year showed a mean change in HbA$_{1c}$

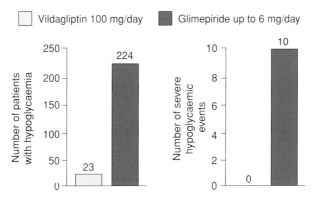

Figure 5.3 Incidence and severity of hypoglycaemic events with vildagliptin and glimepiride during the 52-week treatment period. Reproduced from Ferrannini *et al.* (2009) with permission from Wiley-Blackwell.

from baseline to endpoint of -0.4% in vildagliptin plus metformin-treated patients and -0.5% in glimepiride plus metformin-treated patients, establishing non-inferiority of vildagliptin to glimepiride as add-on to metformin (Ferrannini *et al.*, 2009). No weight gain occurred in vildagliptin-treated patients in contrast to those receiving glimepiride, resulting in a significant between-group difference of 1.79 kg at the end of the study. Vildagliptin was also associated with a tenfold lower incidence of hypoglycaemia than glimepiride: 23 (1.7%) versus 224 (16.2%) of patients presenting with at least one hypoglycaemic event, with no reports of severe events compared with 10 severe hypoglycaemic events in the glimepiride group (Figure 5.3).

Vildagliptin-treated patients did not demonstrate weight gain in any of the above studies and the risk of hypoglycaemia for vildagliptin as add-on to metformin was very low and comparable with placebo and no episodes of severe hypoglycaemia were recorded.

Saxagliptin

Six pivotal Phase 3 trials have reported on the efficacy of saxagliptin as monotherapy, as well as in combination with metformin, sulphonylureas and thiazolidinediones at saxagliptin doses of 2.5, 5, and 10 mg (Table 5.4).

The efficacy of saxagliptin as monotherapy was studied in two 24-week, double-blind, placebo-controlled trials. In treatment-naïve patients, once-daily saxagliptin monotherapy for 24 weeks demonstrated clinically significant reductions in HbA$_{1c}$, fasting and postprandial plasma glucose at all doses compared with placebo (Rosenstock *et al.*, 2009). In a second monotherapy study the efficacy of initial combination therapy with saxagliptin and metformin was compared with saxagliptin and metformin monotherapy in treatment-naïve type 2 diabetes patients with inadequate glycaemic control (Jadzinsky *et al.*, 2009). Saxagliptin in combination with metformin as initial

Table 5.4 HbA$_{1c}$-lowering efficacy of saxagliptin in combination with other antidiabetes agents

Saxagliptin trial	Treatments	Duration (weeks)	Baseline HbA$_{1c}$ (%)	Mean change from baseline HbA$_{1c}$ (%)	Mean difference from comparator (%)
Defronzo et al., 2009	Saxagliptin 2.5 mg + metformin	24	8.1	−0.59	−0.73
	Saxagliptin 5.0 mg + metformin		8.1	−0.69	−0.83
	Saxagliptin 10 mg + metformin		8.0	−0.58	−0.72
	Placebo + metformin		8.1	0.13	
Hollander et al., 2009	Saxagliptin 2.5 mg + thiazolidinedione	24	8.3	−0.66	−0.36
	Saxagliptin 5.0 mg + thiazolidinedione		8.4	−0.94	−0.63
	Placebo + thiazolidinedione		8.2	−0.30	
Chacra et al., 2009	Saxagliptin 2.5 mg + glibenclamide 7.5 mg	24	8.4	−0.54	−0.62
	Saxagliptin 5.0 mg + glibenclamide 7.5 mg		8.5	−0.64	−0.72
	Glibenclamide 10 mg		8.4	0.08	

therapy led to statistically significant improvements compared with either treatment alone across all glycaemic parameters with a tolerability profile similar to the monotherapy components.

In a 24-week combination study with metformin, the addition of saxagliptin 2.5 mg, 5 mg or 10 mg daily resulted in statistically significant reductions in HbA$_{1c}$ from baseline by a mean of 0.7%, 0.8% and 0.7%, respectively, compared with addition of placebo (DeFronzo et al., 2009). Over the 24-week period, saxagliptin also produced significantly greater reductions than placebo in fasting and postprandial plasma glucose levels.

Randomized trials have also been conducted to examine the efficacy of saxagliptin in conjunction with a thiazolidinedione or a sulphonylurea in patients with inadequate glycaemic control on thiazolidinedione or sulphonylurea monotherapy, respectively. In a 24-week study, patients with HbA$_{1c}$ levels of 7.0−10.5% despite stable monotherapy with pioglitazone 30 or 45 mg or rosiglitazone 4 or 8 mg were randomized to treatment with saxagliptin (2.5 or 5 mg) or placebo once daily (Hollander et al., 2009). HbA$_{1c}$, fasting plasma glucose and postprandial plasma glucose were all statistically significantly reduced with the two saxagliptin doses in combination with a thiazolidinedione compared with treatment with a thiazolidinedione in combination with placebo. Similarly, a 24-week study of saxagliptin 2.5 mg or 5 mg addition to submaximal glibenclamide treatment was statistically superior to continued monotherapy with higher doses of the sulphonylurea (Chacra *et al.*, 2009).The weight and hypoglycaemia benefits of DPP-4 inhibitors in general were also reported with saxagliptin in the various clinical trials.

DPP-4 inhibitor safety and tolerability

Both preclinical and clinical experience with DPP-4 inhibitors, although still limited, show that they have good tolerability and few side-effects. A systematic review and meta-analysis of randomized controlled trials with an incretin therapy up to a cut-off point of May 2007 concluded that the available DPP-4 inhibitors (sitagliptin and vildagliptin) were overall very well tolerated, with low absolute rates of adverse events (Amori, Lau and Pittas, 2007). There was no difference in reported mild to moderate hypoglycaemia between DPP-4 inhibitors and comparator group (1.6% vs 1.4%, respectively; risk ratio 1.0, 95% CI 0.5−1.9). In addition, no greater risk of gastrointestinal adverse effects (nausea, vomiting, diarrhoea, and abdominal pain) was reported compared with placebo.

Potential side-effects of DPP-4 inhibition may result from the inadvertent inhibition of related enzymes (DPP-8 and DPP-9) and there is some concern over the role of DPP-4 activity for normal immune function. In two meta-analyses, DPP-4 inhibitors were associated with a slightly increased risk of infection (nasopharyngitis and urinary tract infection) (Amori *et al.*, 2007; Monami *et al.*, 2009), although a pooled analysis of 12 large, double-blind, studies with sitagliptin of up to two years duration found no meaningful differences between sitagliptin and comparator groups in the incidence rate, severity, and type of infections (Williams-Herman *et al.*, 2008). Although data for saxagliptin are more limited, the side-effect profile of this agent appears to be similar to sitagliptin and vildagliptin with a low risk of hypoglycaemia except when coadministered with a sulphonylurea, and a slightly increased risk of respiratory and urinary infections. However, for all of these agents, our understanding of the adverse-event profile is for the most part currently limited to the Phase 3 clinical data, and the long-term safety of prolonged DPP-4 inhibition in patients with type 2 diabetes is unknown.

DPP-4 inhibitor advantages and disadvantages

The secretion of GLP-1 is impaired in patients with type 2 diabetes and as DPP-4 inhibitors can only increase levels of endogenous GLP-1 there is a limit to the levels of active GLP-1 that can be achieved. Furthermore the increases are physiological and fluctuate up and down with meals. As a result of this, HbA_{1c} reductions are slightly less than observed with the incretin mimetics and may not offer sufficient control for patients with inadequate glycaemic control or long-standing type 2 diabetes. Furthermore, the effect of the DPP-4 inhibitors on appetite, food intake and gastric emptying is weak or absent.

Additional studies are also needed to define the long-term efficacy and safety profiles of the DPP-4 inhibitors.

Compared with the incretin mimetics, DPP-4 inhibitors have the advantage of being administered orally and because the increased levels of active GLP-1 observed with the use of DPP-4 inhibitors remain within the physiological range they are associated with a low risk of gastrointestinal side-effects (nausea and vomiting). Unless combined with a sulphonylurea, the DPP-4 inhibitors are associated with a low risk of hypoglycaemia, even in the fasting state or if a meal is missed, consistent with their glucose-dependent mechanism of action. As a class, the DPP-4 inhibitors have a very low potential for drug interactions as they do not inhibit or induce the cytochrome oxidase enzymes. DPP-4 inhibitors can be taken with or without food, produce no weight gain and may have long-term beneficial effects on beta-cell function and mass although so far this has only been demonstrated in animal models.

DPP-4 inhibitor current indications

In the most recent NICE guidelines on 'Type 2 diabetes: newer agents for blood glucose control in type 2 diabetes', sitagliptin or vildagliptin can be considered for dual therapy with either metformin or a sulphonylurea when a patients' glycaemic control is inadequate after treatment with metformin or sulphonylurea monotherapy, and either of the latter drugs is contraindicated or not tolerated (NICE, 2009). Due to the lower risk for hypoglycaemia associated with the DPP-4 inhibitors and thiazolidinediones, they are also recommended for second-line therapy instead of a sulphonylurea if a patient is at severe risk for hypoglycaemia or where hypoglycaemia has to be avoided at all costs. As sitagliptin is licensed for triple therapy it can also be considered with metformin and a sulphonylurea instead of insulin when glycaemic control is inadequate (HbA$_{1c}$ of at least 7.5%) if insulin is unacceptable or inappropriate (e.g. because of employment, or issues related to hypoglycaemia or obesity).

Sitagliptin

In Europe, the three available DPP-4 inhibitors differ slightly in their therapeutic indications. Sitagliptin currently has the widest indications and at a dose of 100 mg once daily is licensed as monotherapy in patients inadequately controlled by diet and exercise alone and for whom metformin is inappropriate, as dual oral therapy in combination with metformin, a sulphonylurea, or a thiazolidinedione, and as triple oral therapy in combination with a sulphonylurea and metformin or a thiazolidinedione and metformin. Sitagliptin is also indicated as add-on to insulin (with or without metformin) when diet and exercise plus stable dosage of insulin do not provide adequate glycaemic control (Januvia SmPC, 2009). A fixed combination of sitagliptin with metformin is also available in Europe.

Vildagliptin

Vildagliptin is approved as a 50 mg dose taken either once or twice daily in combination with metformin, a thiazolidinedione or a sulphonylurea. When used in combination with metformin or a thiazolidinedione the dose is taken as one 50 mg dose in the morning and one 50 mg dose in the evening. When used in dual combination with a sulphonylurea, the recommended dose of vildagliptin is 50 mg once daily administered in the morning. Vildagliptin is not currently licensed for triple therapy with metformin and a sulphonylurea or in combination with insulin (Galvus SmPC, 2009). In Europe, a fixed-dose combination of vildagliptin and metformin also exists.

Saxagliptin

Saxagliptin has the same therapeutic indications as vildagliptin and at a dose of 5 mg once daily is approved for use in combination with metformin, a thiazolidinedione or a sulphonylurea. The safety and efficacy of saxagliptin as triple oral therapy or in combination with insulin has not been established (Onglyza SmPC, 2009).

Place in therapy of the DPP-4 inhibitors

Although slightly less than observed with the incretin mimetics, the DPP-4 inhibitors offer clinically meaningful reductions in HbA_{1c} without significant risk of hypoglycaemia and without causing weight gain. They also have the advantage of being administered orally and with fewer gastrointestinal side-effects than the incretin mimetics. The DPP-4 inhibitors appear most promising as a second-line therapy in combination with metformin, where they are associated with sustained reductions in HbA_{1c} that are equivalent to those achieved with other second-line agents commonly used in combination with metformin, but without the side-effects typically associated with these agents such as weight gain (thiazolidinediones and sulphonylureas) and an increased risk of hypoglycaemia (sulphonylureas). The availability of a DPP-4-inhibitor and metformin in a single-tablet is also likely to increase compliance with this combination. Populations most likely to benefit are those who are overweight or obese, those in whom hypoglycaemia must be avoided at all costs and the elderly. DPP-4 inhibitors may be particularly suitable in the elderly because of their ease of use, a low potential for drug:drug interactions and their favourable tolerability profile.

References

Amori RE, Lau J, Pittas AG. (2007) Efficacy and safety of incretin therapy in type 2 diabetes: systematic review and meta-analysis. *JAMA*; 298:194–206.

Aschner P, Kipnes MS, Lunceford JK, *et al.* (2006) Effect of the dipeptidyl peptidase-4 inhibitor sitagliptin as monotherapy on glycemic control in patients with type 2 diabetes. *Diabetes Care*; 29:2632–2637.

Bolli G, Dotta F, Rochotte E, Cohen SE. (2008) Efficacy and tolerability of vildagliptin vs. piogitazone when added to metformin: a 24-week, randomized, double-blind study. *Diabetes Obes Metab*; 10:82–90.

Bosi E, Camisasca RP, Collober C, *et al.* (2007) Effects of vildagliptin on glucose control over 24 weeks in patients with type 2 diabetes inadequately controlled with metformin. *Diabetes Care*; 30:890–895.

Chacra AR, Tan GH, Apanovitch A, *et al.*; CV181-040 Investigators (2009) Saxagliptin added to a submaximal dose of sulphonylurea improves glycaemic control compared with up-titration of sulphonylurea in patients with type 2 diabetes: a randomised controlled trial. *Int J Clin Pract*; 63:1395–1406.

Charbonnel B, Karasik A, Liu J, *et al.* (2006) Efficacy and safety of the dipeptidyl peptidase-4 inhibitor sitagliptin added to ongoing metformin therapy in patients with type 2 diabetes inadequately controlled with metformin alone. *Diabetes Care*; 29:2638–2643.

Deacon CF, Holst JJ. (2006) Dipeptidyl peptidase IV inhibitors: a promising new therapeutic approach for the management of type 2 diabetes. *Int J Biochem Cell Biol*; 38:831–844.

DeFronzo RA, Hissa MN, Garber AJ, *et al.*; Saxagliptin 014 Study Group (2009) The efficacy and safety of saxagliptin when added to metformin therapy in patients with inadequately controlled type 2 diabetes with metformin alone. *Diabetes Care*; 32:1649–1655.

Dejager S, Razac S, Foley JE, Schweizer A. (2007) Vildagliptin in drug-naïve patients with type 2 diabetes: a 24-week, double-blind, randomized, placebo-controlled, multiple-dose study. *Horm Metab Res*; 39:218–223.

Ferrannini E, Fonseca V, Zinman B, *et al.* (2009) Fifty-two-week efficacy and safety of vildagliptin vs. glimepiride in patients with type 2 diabetes mellitus inadequately controlled on metformin monotherapy. *Diabetes Obes Metab*; 11:157–166.

Fonseca V, Schweizer A, Albrecht D, *et al.* (2007) Addition of vildagliptin to insulin improves glycaemic control in type 2 diabetes. *Diabetologia*; 50:1148–1155.

Galvus SmPC (2009) Novartis Pharmaceuticals UK Ltd. Galvus 50 mg tablets. Summary of Product Characteristics (UK), August 2009. Available at: http://emc.medicines.org.uk/medicine/20734/SPC/Galvus+50+mg+Tablets

Garber AJ, Schweizer A, Baron MA, *et al.* (2007) Vildagliptin in combination with piogitazone improves glycaemic control in patients with type 2 diabetes failing thiazolidinedione monotherapy: a randomized, placebo-controlled study. *Diabetes Obes Metab*; 9:166–174.

Garber AJ, Foley JE, Banerji MA, *et al.* (2008) Effects of vildagliptin on glucose control in patients with type 2 diabetes inadequately controlled with a sulphonylurea. *Diabetes Obes Metab*; 10:1047–1056.

Goldstein B, Feinglos MN, Lunceford JK, *et al.*; Sitagliptin 036 Study Group (2007) Effect of initial combination therapy with sitagliptin, a dipeptidyl peptidase-4 inhibitor, and metformin on glycemic control in patients with type 2 diabetes. *Diabetes Care*; 30:1979–1987.

Hollander P, Li J, Allen E, Chen R; CV181-013 Investigators (2009) Saxagliptin added to a thiazolidinedione improves glycemic control in patients with type 2 diabetes and inadequate control on thiazolidinedione alone. *J Clin Endocrinol Metab*; 94:4810–4819.

Jadzinsky M, Pfützner A, Paz-Pacheco E, *et al.*; CV181-039 Investigators (2009) Saxagliptin given in combination with metformin as initial therapy improves glycaemic control in patients with type 2 diabetes compared with either monotherapy: a randomized controlled trial. *Diabetes Obes Metab*; 11:611–622.

Januvia SmPC (2009) Merck Sharp & Dohme Limited. JANUVIA 100 mg film-coated tablets. Summary of Product Characteristics (UK), November 2009. Available at: http://emc.medicines.org.uk/medicine/19609#INDICATIONS

Monami M, Iacomelli I, Marchionni N, Mannucci E. (2010) Dipeptydil peptidase-4 inhibitors in type 2 diabetes: A meta-analysis of randomized clinical trials. *Nutr Metab Cardiovasc Dis*; 20:224–235.

National Institute for Health and Clinical Excellence (NICE) (2009) Type 2 diabetes: newer agents for blood glucose control. NICE short clinical guidelines 87. Available from: http://www.nice.org.uk/nicemedia/pdf/CG87NICEGuideline.pdf. Last accessed February 2010.

Nauck MA, Meininger G, Sheng D, *et al.* (2007) Efficacy and safety of the dipeptidyl peptidase-4 inhibitor, sitagliptin, compared with the sulfonylurea, glipizide, in patients with type 2 diabetes inadequately controlled on metformin alone: a randomized, double-blind, non-inferiority trial. *Diabetes Obes Metab*; 9:194–205.

Onglyza SmPC (2009) Bristol Myers Squibb/AstraZeneca EEIG. Onglyza 5 mg film-coated tablets. Summary of Product Characteristics (UK), October 2009. Available at: http://emc.medicines.org.uk/medicine/22315/SPC/Onglyza+5mg+film-coated+tablets

Pi-Sunyer FX, Schweizer A, Mills D, Dejager S. (2007) Efficacy and tolerability of vildagliptin monotherapy in drug-naïve patients with type 2 diabetes. *Diabetes Res Clin Pract*; 76:132–138.

Raz I, Hanefeld M, Xu L, *et al.* (2006) Efficacy and safety of the dipeptidyl peptidase-4 inhibitor sitagliptin as monotherapy in patients with type 2 diabetes mellitus. *Diabetologia*; 49:2564–2571.

Rosenstock J, Fitchet M. (2008) Vildagliptin: clinical trials programme in monotherapy and combination therapy for type 2 diabetes. *Int J Clin Pract*; 62(Suppl 159):15–23.

Rosenstock J, Brazg R, Andryuk PJ, *et al.* (2006) Efficacy and safety of the dipeptidyl peptidase-4 inhibitor sitagliptin added to ongoing pioglitazone therapy in patients with type 2 diabetes: a 24-week, multicenter, randomized, double-blind, placebo-controlled, parallel-group study. *Clin Ther*; 28:1556–1568.

Rosenstock J, Baron MA, Dejager S, *et al.* (2007a) Comparison of vildagliptin and rosiglitazone monotherapy in patients with type 2 diabetes: a 24-week, double-blind, randomized trial. *Diabetes Care*; 30:217–223.

Rosenstock J, Kim SW, Baron MA, *et al.* (2007b) Efficacy and tolerability of initial combination therapy with vildagliptin and pioglitazone compared with component monotherapy in patients with type 2 diabetes. *Diabetes Obes Metab*; 9:175–185.

Rosenstock J, Aguilar-Salinas C, Klein E, *et al.*; CV181-011 Study Investigators (2009) Effect of saxagliptin monotherapy in treatment-naïve patients with type 2 diabetes. *Curr Med Res Opin*; 25:2401–2411.

Schweizer A, Couturier A, Foley JE, Dejager S. (2007) Comparison between vildagliptin and metformin to sustain reductions in HbA(1c) over 1 year in drug-naïve patients with type 2 diabetes. *Diabet Med*; 24:955–961.

Williams-Herman D, Round E, Swern AS, *et al.* (2008) Safety and tolerability of sitagliptin in patients with type 2 diabetes: a pooled analysis. *BMC Endocr Disord*; 8:14.

6 Sodium-glucose Cotransporter-2 Inhibitors

The kidneys play a central role in the regulation of plasma glucose levels and have recently become a new target for the treatment of type 2 diabetes with the development of the sodium-glucose cotransporter-2 (SGLT-2) inhibitors. Blood glucose in the circulation is continuously filtered in the glomeruli of the kidneys and then reabsorbed by active transport mechanisms in the renal proximal convoluted tubules, a process that normally prevents the loss of glucose in the urine. The first step in the reabsorption of glucose from the urine involves the transport of glucose from the glomerular filtrate into the proximal tubule epithelial cells, a process that is accomplished by two sodium-glucose cotransporters: SGLT-1 and SGLT-2 (White, 2010). SGLT-1 is the main transporter for glucose absorption in the gastrointestinal tract, but in the kidney it is less significant accounting for about 10% of glucose reabsorption. SGLT-2 is expressed exclusively in the S1 segment of the proximal tubule and accounts for about 90% of renal glucose reabsorption, properties that have made it a promising target for drug development and the focus of significant research.

Early observations with the natural SGLT-inhibitor phlorizin revealed that inhibition of renal and intestinal glucose transport was able to improve control of diabetes in animal models, although this non-selective inhibitor was unsuitable for clinical development (Rossetti *et al.*, 1987). Further evidence for the viability of this approach has come from studies of people with familial renal glucosuria, a condition in which urinary glucose loss is increased, but which otherwise has no known long-term adverse consequences for health (van den Heuvel *et al.*, 2002). Findings such as this have improved our understanding of the physiology of renal glucose transport and facilitated the development of drugs that selectively target the SGLT-2 cotransporter. These agents block glucose and sodium from being reabsorbed resulting in increased renal excretion of glucose. By reducing fasting and postprandial plasma glucose without causing hypoglycaemia the SGLT-2 inhibitors may offer a unique insulin-independent method of reducing levels of high blood glucose in patients with diabetes (Ehrenkranz *et al.*, 2005). A number of SGLT-2 inhibitors

New Mechanisms in Glucose Control, First Edition. Anthony H. Barnett & Jenny Grice.
© 2011 Anthony H. Barnett & Jenny Grice. Published 2011 Blackwell Publishing Ltd.

are in clinical development. The most advanced is dapagliflozin, which is currently in Phase 3 clinical trials.

Dapagliflozin

Dapagliflozin is a highly selective SGLT-2 inhibitor with 1000 x selectivity over SGLT-1, as a result of which there is no interference with SGLT-1-mediated intestinal glucose absorption (Meng *et al.*, 2008). After oral administration, dapagliflozin is rapidly absorbed with a median time to maximum plasma concentration of one hour (Komoroski *et al.*, 2009a). When administered at doses of 5–100 mg/day, dapagliflozin increases urinary glucose excretion to 37–70 mg/day over 24 hours compared with no change with placebo in healthy subjects and in patients with type 2 diabetes (Komoroski *et al.*, 2009a; Komoroski *et al.*, 2009b).

In a Phase 2 study, 47 patients with type 2 diabetes were randomized to dapagliflozin 5 mg, 25 mg, or 100 mg, or placebo for 14 days (Komoroski *et al.*, 2009b). Significant reductions in fasting serum glucose of 9.3% were observed on Day 2 with 100 mg dapagliflozin. At the end of the study, significant reductions in fasting serum glucose were achieved with all doses compared with placebo: 11.7% (5 mg), 13.3% (25 mg) and 21.8% (100 mg) (Komoroski *et al.*, 2009b). All dapagliflozin doses also produced significant improvements in oral glucose tolerance test from Day 2 compared with placebo indicating benefits on postprandial plasma glucose.

In a Phase 2 dose-ranging study, 389 treatment-naïve patients with type 2 diabetes were randomly assigned to one of five dapagliflozin doses, metformin extended release, or placebo for 12 weeks (List *et al.*, 2009). The patients studied were typical of those with type 2 diabetes of recent onset, and averaged about 58 years of age with a baseline HbA_{1c} level ranging from 7.7–8.0%. All doses of dapagliflozin produced increases in urinary glucose of 52–85 g/day and were associated with reductions in HbA_{1c} of 0.55–0.90%, which were statistically significant compared with placebo (Figure 6.1). Reductions in fasting plasma glucose of 0.9–1.7 mmol/L were observed across the dapagliflozin arms as well as a weight loss of 1.3–2.0 kg compared with placebo, which corresponds to a reduction in body weight of 2.5–3.4% with dapagliflozin (Figure 6.2).

A 12-week pilot study has evaluated dapagliflozin 10 mg and 20 mg in insulin-resistant patients not achieving adequate glycaemic control with insulin and oral antidiabetes agents (metformin and/or thiazolidinediones) (Wilding *et al.*, 2009). At the end of the study, greater reductions in HbA_{1c}, postprandial plasma glucose and body weight were observed with dapagliflozin compared with placebo. Reductions in HbA_{1c} ranged from 0.61–0.69% in the two dapagliflozin-treatment arms, compared with a 0.09% increase in the placebo arm. Importantly, dapagliflozin appeared to counteract the weight gain associated with insulin treatment. Weight loss in the

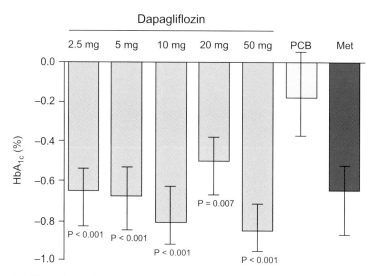

Figure 6.1 Mean change from baseline HbA$_{1c}$ with dapagliflozin. PCB, placebo; MET, metformin. Reproduced from List *et al.* (2009) with permission from the American Diabetes Association. © 2009 American Diabetes Association.

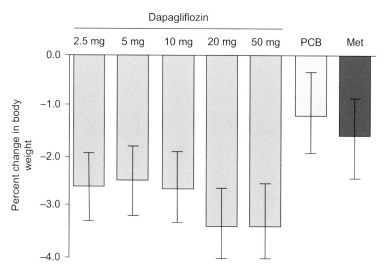

Figure 6.2 Adjusted mean (95% CI) percent change from baseline in body weight after 12 weeks of dapagliflozin treatment. Reproduced from List *et al.* (2009) with permission from the American Diabetes Association. © 2009 American Diabetes Association.

dapagliflozin group ranged from 4.3−4.5 kg compared with a 1.9 kg loss for placebo.

In a Phase 3 study, 546 patients not achieving adequate glycaemic control with metformin (at least 1500 mg/day) were randomized to adjunctive oral dapagliflozin 2.5 mg, 5 mg, 10 mg or placebo once daily for 24 weeks (Bailey *et al.*, 2010). Mean HbA$_{1c}$ reductions from baseline were −0.67%, −0.70% and −0.84% (all P < 0.001) in the dapagliflozin 2.5 mg, 5 mg, and 10 mg groups, respectively, compared with −0.30% in the placebo group. Patients assigned to placebo lost a mean of 0.9 kg compared with 2.2 kg with dapagliflozin 2.5 mg, 3 kg with dapagliflozin 5 mg, and 2.9 kg with dapagliflozin 10 mg. Symptoms of hypoglycaemia occurred in similar proportions of patients in the dapagliflozin and placebo groups (approximately 3%). In addition to dapagliflozin, a number of other SGLT-2 inhibitors are in development, the most advanced of which is canagliflozin. However, at the time of writing no published papers were available on this agent. The clinical development of two agents, sergliflozin etabonate and remogliflozin etabonate, was halted at Phase 2 trials.

Safety and tolerability

The side-effect profile of the SGLT-2 inhibitors is likely to depend on the ability to selectively inhibit SGLT-2 over SGLT-1, given that SGLT-1 inhibition is associated with glucose malabsorption and diarrhoea. To date, short-term safety data with the SGLT-2 inhibitors indicate that these agents appear well tolerated with no major difference in adverse events across treatment groups (Komoroski *et al.*, 2009a; Komoroski *et al.*, 2009b; List *et al.*, 2009). The only exception is a higher incidence of genitourinary infections compared with placebo (Table 6.1) (Bailey *et al.*, 2010; List *et al.*, 2009). It is likely that the higher glucose concentrations in the urine may allow yeast organisms to flourish. The increase in urinary glucose excretion is not associated with a greater risk of hypoglycaemia or excessive losses of serum electrolytes and despite the increased urinary volume, few patients complain of excessive urination. The long-term safety of these agents is not yet known.

Table 6.1 Most common adverse events occurring with dapagliflozin therapy.

Most common adverse events (%)	Dapagliflozin (2.5−50 mg)	Metformin extended release	Placebo
Urinary tract infections	5−12	7	6
Genital infections	2−7	2	0
Hypoglycaemia	6−10	9	4
Nausea	3−7	11	6
Headache	2−7	4	11
Diarrhoea	2−7	13	7

Adapted from List *et al.* (2009).

SGLT-2 inhibitor advantages and disadvantages

An increase in urinary tract infections and vaginitis has been observed in trials with the SGLT-2 inhibitors and may be a potential drawback of increased urinary glucose excretion. Safety data are also required in relation to long-term use and drug interactions. Although SGLT-2 inhibitors do not directly target the pathophysiology of type 2 diabetes they have an advantage in that the beneficial effects on glycaemic parameters associated with increasing urinary glucose loss are achieved with a net energy deficit, promoting weight loss. In addition, these agents are oral and as they do not affect glucose counter-regulatory mechanisms they are associated with a low risk of hypoglycaemia. The diuretic effect may also be an advantage in patients with congestive heart failure. The unique mechanism of action of the SGLT-2 inhibitors, which is independent of insulin secretion or insulin resistance, suggests that these agents may still be effective in patients with advance beta-cell dysfunction or severe insulin resistance. They will also complement therapy with existing oral antidiabetes agents or insulin.

References

Bailey CJ, Gross JL, Pieters A, *et al.* (2010) Effect of dapagliflozin in patients with type 2 diabetes who have inadequate glycaemic control with metformin: a randomised, double-blind, placebo-controlled trial. *Lancet*; 375:2223–2233.

Ehrenkranz JR, Lewis NG, Kahn CR, Roth J. (2005) Phlorizin: a review. *Diabetes Metab Res Rev*; 21:31–38.

Komoroski B, Vachharajani N, Boulton D, *et al.* (2009a) Dapagliflozin, a novel SGLT2 inhibitor, induces dose-dependent glucosuria in healthy subjects. *Clin Pharmacol Ther*; 85:520–526.

Komoroski B, Vachharajani N, Feng Y, *et al.* (2009b) Dapagliflozin, a novel, selective SGLT2 inhibitor, improved glycemic control over 2 weeks in patients with type 2 diabetes mellitus. *Clin Pharmacol Ther*; 85:513–519.

List JF, Woo V, Morales E, *et al.* (2009) Sodium-glucose cotransport inhibition with dapagliflozin in type 2 diabetes. *Diabetes Care*; 32:650–657.

Meng W, Ellsworth BA, Nirschl AA, *et al.* (2008) Discovery of dapagliflozin: a potent, selective renal sodium-dependent glucose cotransporter 2 (SGLT2) inhibitor for the treatment of type 2 diabetes. *J Med Chem*; 51:1145–1149.

Rossetti L, Smith D, Shulman GI, *et al.* (1987) Correction of hyperglycemia with phlorizin normalizes tissue sensitivity to insulin in diabetic rats. *J Clin Invest*; 79:1510–1515.

van den Heuvel LP, Assink K, Willemsen M, Monnens L. (2002) Autosomal recessive renal glucosuria attributable to a mutation in the sodium glucose cotransporter (SGLT2). *Hum Genet*; 111:544–547.

White JR. (2010) Apple trees to sodium glucose co-transporter inhibitors: a review of SGLT2 inhibition. *Clin Diabetes*; 28:5–10.

Wilding JP, Norwood P, T'joen C, *et al.* (2009) A study of dapagliflozin in patients with type 2 diabetes receiving high doses of insulin plus insulin sensitizers: applicability of a novel insulin-independent treatment. *Diabetes Care*; 32:1656–1662.

7 | Pipeline Diabetes Therapies

The complexity of glucose metabolism and the number of cellular processes affected by diabetes provide ample opportunity for the development of new drug targets and first-in-class molecules (Table 7.1).

Taspoglutide

Taspoglutide is a glucagon-like peptide 1 (GLP-1) receptor agonist with 93% homology to endogenous GLP-1 and is currently in Phase 3 trials. When administered as a once-weekly subcutaneous injection to people with type 2 diabetes, plasma concentrations of the drug peak within 24 hours after injection and are associated with significant reductions in fasting and postprandial plasma glucose compared with placebo for up to 14 days after the initial injection (Kapitza *et al.*, 2009). In an eight-week, dose-ranging study in patients with type 2 diabetes inadequately controlled with metformin alone, all doses of taspoglutide achieved significantly greater reductions in HbA_{1c} compared with patients receiving placebo plus metformin (Nauck *et al.*, 2009). The mean decrease in HbA_{1c} of 1.1% from a baseline of 7.9 compares favourably with available GLP-1-receptor agonists. Taspoglutide also produced a progressive and dose-dependent weight loss. Similar to other GLP-1 receptor agonists, the most frequent adverse event with taspoglutide treatment was mild-to-moderate nausea. Unfortunately, further development of this agent has been (temporarily?) suspended because of hypersensitivity reactions in some patients.

Linagliptin

Linagliptin is a dipeptidyl peptidase-4 (DPP-4) inhibitor in Phase 3 development for the treatment of type 2 diabetes with a long duration of action making it suitable for once-daily dosing (Heise *et al.*, 2009). The Phase 3 programme with linagliptin comprises five pivotal trials, which are evaluating the efficacy and safety of linagliptin alone and in combination with commonly used diabetes treatments including metformin, sulphonylureas and

New Mechanisms in Glucose Control, First Edition. Anthony H. Barnett & Jenny Grice.
© 2011 Anthony H. Barnett & Jenny Grice. Published 2011 Blackwell Publishing Ltd.

Table 7.1 Pipeline therapies for type 2 diabetes

Pipeline therapy	Mechanism of action	Stage of development
Taspoglutide	GLP-1 receptor agonist	Phase 3
Linagliptin	DPP-4 inhibitor	Phase 3
Bile acid receptor agonists	Activate TGR-5 to increase energy expenditure and secretion of GLP-1	Phase 2
Glucokinase activators	Increase sensitivity of glucokinase to glucose promoting insulin secretion and increasing hepatic glucose uptake	Phase 2
Sirtuins	Stimulate mitochondrial activity in metabolically active tissues	Phase 2
Sodium-glucose cotransporter-1 inhibitors	Decrease intestinal glucose absorption	Phase 1
Sodium-glucose cotransporter-2 antisense inhibitors	Inhibit expression of the SGLT-2 gene	Phase 1
GIP agonists	Glucose-dependent insulin secretion	Preclinical
GIP antagonists	Reversal of obesity-related metabolic disturbances	Preclinical
Glucagon receptor antagonists	Prevent glucagon from stimulating hepatic glucose output	Preclinical

thiazolidinediones. Data from a 12-week Phase 2 study in 333 patients failing to achieve glycaemic control despite being treated with metformin, showed statistically significant reductions in HbA_{1c}, with placebo-corrected reductions from baseline of 0.73% and 0.67% for linagliptin 5 mg and 10 mg, respectively (Forst *et al.*, 2010). In this study, the incidence of adverse events was similar to placebo. At the time of writing, data from only one of the pivotal Phase 3 trials have been published. In this trial, 700 patients inadequately controlled on a maximum tolerated dose of metformin monotherapy were randomized to linagliptin 5 mg (n = 523) or placebo (n = 177) (Taskinen *et al.*, 2011). After 24 weeks of treatment, the difference in mean change from baseline HbA_{1c} was −0.64% compared with placebo (P < 0.0001). Linagliptin was also associated with significantly greater reductions in both fasting and postprandial plasma glucose. The drug had no influence on body weight and was well tolerated. In contrast to other DPP-4 inhibitors, only a minor fraction of linagliptin is eliminated through the kidneys, which may be an advantage in patients with renal impairment.

Bile acid receptor agonists

Bile acids are known to be key regulators of lipid, glucose and overall energy metabolism and bile acid activation of the G protein-coupled receptor

TGR5 has been shown to induce energy expenditure in muscle and brown fat and control the secretion of GLP-1 (Thomas *et al.*, 2009). A modified human bile acid has been developed, INT-777, which acts as a selective TGR5 agonist. In animal models this agent increases energy expenditure in muscle and brown fat thereby reducing fat mass, and improves glycaemic parameters via dual effects on energy expenditure and increased GLP-1 secretion. The agent is currently in Phase 2 trials.

Glucokinase activators

Glucokinase is the enzyme responsible for phosphorylating glucose to glucose-6 phosphate and is expressed in pancreatic beta cells and liver cells. As blood glucose levels rise after a meal, the enzyme acts as a sensor for glucose-stimulated insulin release in beta cells and in the liver glucokinase phosphorylation of glucose promotes glycogen synthesis, increasing hepatic glucose uptake and decreasing hepatic glucose production. In animal models, activators of glucokinase increase the sensitivity of the enzyme to glucose, leading to increased insulin secretion and liver glycogen synthesis and a decrease in liver glucose output (Coope *et al.*, 2006). Potential concerns include hypoglycaemia due to increased insulin secretion. However, liver-selective glucokinase activators with lower potential for hypoglycaemia have also been developed and tested in preclinical models (Bebernitz *et al.*, 2009). A number of glucokinase activators are in development and have progressed to clinical trials.

Sirtuins

The SIRT1 enzyme is the most well studied of the seven human sirtuin family members. It is involved in regulating key cellular processes, notably the efficiency and number of mitochondria, and is emerging as a major therapeutic target for the treatment of type 2 diabetes as well as other diseases. Activators of SIRT1 have been shown to stimulate mitochondrial activity in metabolically active tissues, such as muscle, increasing metabolic rate, driving glucose metabolism, and thereby improving insulin sensitivity. These agents have demonstrated improved metabolic function in animal models of diabetes and obesity, suggesting that they may have therapeutic potential in type 2 diabetes. Development of these molecules has progressed to clinical trials with the lead molecule SRT2104 being evaluated in a Phase 2 trial in patients with type 2 diabetes.

Sodium-glucose cotransporter-1 inhibitors

Sodium-glucose cotransporter-1 (SGLT-1) is abundant in the small intestine and plays a major role in glucose absorption from the gut. It is also found in the brain, skeletal and heart muscle, liver, lungs and kidneys. Preclinical studies in rodent models of diabetes have shown that SGLT-1 inhibitors improve postprandial hyperglycaemia by decreasing intestinal glucose absorption (Kumeda *et al.*, 2007). The lead agents are currently in Phase 1 trials.

Sodium-glucose cotransporter-2 antisense inhibitors

In addition to the sodium-glucose cotransporter-2 (SGLT-2) inhibitors, a novel approach to target SGLT-2 uses an RNAase H chimeric antisense oligonucleotide to inhibit the expression of the SGLT-2 gene *in vivo*. Preclinical studies with ISIS 388626, as yet only published in abstract form, demonstrated that the antisense oligonucleotide was able to selectively target the kidney proximal tubules, with no accumulation in other tissues, and reduce SGLT-2 expression by up to 80% with once-weekly administration (Wancewicz *et al.*, 2008). In rodent models, there were increases in urinary glucose excretion, improvements in blood glucose control, and HbA$_{1c}$ reductions. A Phase 1 trial to assess the safety and tolerability of ISIS 388626 at single and multiple doses in healthy volunteers is ongoing (Clinical trials.gov).

Glucose-dependent insulinotropic polypeptide agonists and antagonists

Glucose-dependent insulinotropic polypeptide (GIP or gastric inhibitory polypeptide) is an incretin hormone secreted from the small intestine in response to nutrient absorption, which appears to have two main actions. In healthy individuals GIP stimulates insulin release in a glucose-dependent manner, but in patients with type 2 diabetes the effects are diminished. One line of research targeting GIP is therefore focusing on analogues that are resistant to inactivation by the enzyme dipeptidyl peptidase-4 (Irwin and Flatt, 2009).

GIP receptors are also found on adipocytes and appear to be involved in the conversion of excessive amounts of dietary fat into adipocyte tissue stores (Irwin and Flatt, 2009). Given the link between the consumption of energy-rich, high-fat diets and the development of obesity, insulin resistance and type 2 diabetes, GIP receptor antagonism may therefore also be a potential target for the treatment of obesity and insulin resistance. In support of this, both genetic and chemical ablation of GIP signalling in mice with obesity and diabetes can protect against, or even reverse many obesity-associated metabolic disturbances (Irwin and Flatt, 2009). Proof of concept is also provided by the reversal of diabetes in obese people undergoing Roux-en-Y bypass surgery, which involves surgical bypass of GIP-secreting cells in the upper small intestine (Irwin and Flatt, 2009).

Glucagon receptor antagonists

Elevated glucagon levels contribute to hyperglycaemia in type 2 diabetes by inappropriately stimulating hepatic glucose output in both fasting and fed states. Blocking the binding of glucagon to its receptor is therefore a novel approach to reduce plasma glucose levels. In animal models of diabetes glucagon receptor antagonists have demonstrated significant and consistent lowering of blood glucose following oral administration and are currently in preclinical development.

References

Bebernitz GR, Beaulieu V, Dale BA, *et al.* (2009) Investigation of functionally liver selective glucokinase activators for the treatment of type 2 diabetes. *J Med Chem*; 52:6142–6152.

Clinical Trials.gov. Safety, tolerability and activity study of multiple doses of ISIS 388626 in healthy volunteers. Available at: http://clinicaltrials.gov/ct2/show/NCT00836225?term=ISIS+388626. Last accessed February 2010.

Coope GJ, Atkinson AM, Allott C, *et al.* (2006) Predictive blood glucose lowering efficacy by glucokinase activators in high fat fed female Zucker rats. *Br J Pharmacol*; 149:328–335.

Forst T, Uhlig-Laske B, Ring A, *et al.* (2010) Linagliptin (BI 1356), a potent and selective DPP-4 inhibitor, is safe and efficacious in combination with metformin in patients with inadequately controlled Type 2 diabetes. *Diabetic Med*; 27:1409–1419.

Heise T, Graefe-Mody EU, Hüttner S, *et al.* (2009) Pharmacokinetics, pharmacodynamics and tolerability of multiple oral doses of linagliptin, a dipeptidyl peptidase-4 inhibitor in male type 2 diabetes patients. *Diabetes Obes Metab*; 11:786–794.

Irwin N, Flatt PR. (2009) Evidence for beneficial effects of compromised gastric inhibitory polypeptide action in obesity-related diabetes and possible therapeutic implications. *Diabetologia*; 52:1724–1731.

Kapitza C, Heise T, Birman P, *et al.* (2009) Pharmacokinetic and pharmacodynamic properties of taspoglutide, a once-weekly, human GLP-1 analogue, after single-dose administration in patients with type 2 diabetes. *Diabet Med*; 26:1156–1164.

Kumeda S-I, Io F, Kitajima R, *et al.* (2007) Novel SGLT inhibitor (SGL5094) improves postprandial hyperglycemia through the suppression of SGLT1-mediated glucose transport across the small intestine. Program and abstracts of the 67th Scientific Sessions of the American Diabetes Association, June 22–26, 2007; Chicago, Illinois. Abstract 0510-P.

Nauck MA, Ratner RE, Kapitza C, *et al.* (2009) Treatment with the human once-weekly glucagon-like peptide-1 analog taspoglutide in combination with metformin improves glycemic control and lowers body weight in patients with type 2 diabetes inadequately controlled with metformin alone: a double-blind placebo-controlled study. *Diabetes Care*; 32:1237–1243.

Taskinen M-R, Rosenstock J, Tamminen I, *et al.* (2011) Safety and efficacy of linagliptin as add-on therapy to metformin in patients with type 2 diabetes: a randomised, double-blind, placebo-controlled study. *Diabetes Obes Metab*; 13:65–74.

Thomas C, Gioiello A, Noriega L, *et al.* (2009) TGR5-mediated bile acid sensing controls glucose homeostasis. *Cell Metab*; 10:167–177.

Wancewicz EV, Siwkowski A, Meibohm B, *et al.* (2008) Long term safety and efficacy of ISIS 388626, an optimized SGLT2 antisense inhibitor, in multiple diabetic and euglycemic species. Program and abstracts of the 68th Scientific Sessions of the American Diabetes Association, June 6–10, 2008; San Francisco, California. Abstract 334-OR.

8 Bariatric Surgery for the Treatment of Type 2 Diabetes

The health risks associated with obesity are widely recognized. It is an important risk factor for a number of chronic diseases including type 2 diabetes and is also directly related to increased mortality and lower life expectancy (Kopelman, 2010). Intentional weight loss in obese patients as a result of lifestyle, pharmaceutical or surgical interventions for obesity is consistently associated with a reduction in the risk of developing diabetes (Kopelman, 2010). In obese patients already diagnosed with type 2 diabetes, weight loss can result in reduced clinical symptoms and reduced medication. Furthermore, a remarkable finding is that in obese individuals who have undergone surgical intervention to achieve their weight loss, a resolution of diabetes is observed in over 80% of patients (Buchwald *et al.*, 2009; Rubino *et al.*, 2010).

Potential mechanisms of diabetes resolution after bariatric surgery

Bariatric surgery is a very effective treatment for obesity. Approximately one third of obese patients undergoing surgery also have type 2 diabetes (Pinkney and Kerrigan, 2004), and for many of them, an additional benefit of surgery is that their diabetes resolves. A review of the published literature indicates that this occurs in 84—98% of patients after bypass procedures such as Roux-en-Y gastric bypass, and in 48—68% of patients after restrictive procedures such as laparoscopic adjustable gastric banding (Vetter *et al.*, 2009). The fact that glycaemic control improves markedly within days of the surgery suggests that mechanisms other than restriction of calories are involved, the most likely explanation being the effects of an altered pattern of gut hormone secretion after the surgical procedure (Rubino *et al.*, 2010). A number of gut hormones influence insulin sensitivity including the incretin hormones glucagon-like peptide-1 (GLP-1) and glucose-dependent insulinotropic peptide (GIP), secreted by intestinal L and K cells, respectively, in response to nutrients, as well as ghrelin and peptide YY. Surgical procedures that bypass the upper small intestine exclude the duodenum and proximal jejunum, the location of

New Mechanisms in Glucose Control, First Edition. Anthony H. Barnett & Jenny Grice.
© 2011 Anthony H. Barnett & Jenny Grice. Published 2011 Blackwell Publishing Ltd.

Table 8.1 Resolution of diabetes with different weight loss surgical procedures. Patients with condition resolved (%)

	Gastric banding	Gastroplasty	Gastric bypass	Bilipancreatic diversion/duodenal switch	Total
Excess body weight loss	46.2	55.5	59.7	63.6	55.9
Resolved overall	56.7	79.7	80.3	95.1	78.1
Resolved < 2 years	55.0	81.4	81.6	94.0	80.3
Resolved ≥ 2 years	58.3	77.5	70.9	95.9	74.6

Reproduced from Buchwald *et al.* (2009) with permission from Elsevier.

GIP-secreting K-cells and ghrelin-secreting cells, and deliver nutrients directly to the distal small intestine, which enhances secretion of GLP-1 and peptide YY. There is also the possibility that surgery may influence as yet unidentified hormones involved in metabolic control.

Efficacy of bariatric surgery for the treatment of type 2 diabetes

Marked improvements in insulin sensitivity have been observed in bariatric patients within the first few days after gastric bypass procedures and before any weight loss has occurred (Rubino *et al.*, 2010). In a recent meta-analysis of data from 621 studies involving more than 4000 patients with diabetes, complete resolution of diabetes (defined as normoglycaemia with no diabetes medications) occurred in 78.1% of patients (Buchwald *et al.*, 2009). Among studies reporting resolution or improvement of diabetes, 86.6% of patients experienced either outcome. Table 8.1 shows the rates of diabetes resolution for the different bariatric procedures. In this meta-analysis, greater weight loss and shorter duration of diabetes also predicted remission of diabetes (Buchwald *et al.*, 2009).

Despite the impressive nature of these data, only 4.7% of the studies were randomized controlled trials and none of the studies were designed specifically to examine the effects of bariatric surgery as a treatment for diabetes in patients with diabetes. Studies are now ongoing to determine if bariatric surgery, either gastric bypass or adjustable gastric banding, is more effective than intensive lifestyle modification to reduce weight and ultimately treat type 2 diabetes both in people with a body mass index (BMI) over 35 kg/m^2 and in those with a BMI over 30 kg/m^2. However, weight-loss surgery has yet to be compared with medical treatment for weight loss, or against standard medical treatment for diabetes in any randomized controlled trial with diabetes-specific end points. Any future trials should enrol varied patient populations both in terms of diabetes duration and severity, as well as according to age, sex and ethnicity, to determine who the most appropriate candidates for weight loss surgery are.

While there remains a need for long-term randomized controlled trials before bariatric surgery is used more widely as a first-line treatment for obese patients with type 2 diabetes, the existing evidence that weight loss surgery often leads to significant improvement in type 2 diabetes has led many experts to call for a lowering of the BMI recommendation in people who are both overweight and have type 2 diabetes. In the UK, the National Institute for Health and Clinical Excellence (NICE) obesity guidelines currently recommend that bariatric surgery should be reserved for individuals with a BMI of at least 35 kg/m^2 (NICE, 2006). However, in December 2009, Diabetes Surgery Summit delegates issued a consensus statement in which they recognize the value of surgical approaches to treat diabetes in carefully selected patients (Rubino *et al.*, 2009). In this statement, gastric bypass was deemed a reasonable treatment option for patients with poorly controlled diabetes and a BMI of 30 kg/m^2 or more. The statement also highlighted that clinical trials to investigate the exact role of surgery in patients with less severe obesity and diabetes should be considered a priority.

Considerations

Although data for bariatric surgery in people with diabetes are provocative, this evidence comes from patients who have undergone bariatric surgery primarily for other reasons. There is a need for randomized controlled trials to clarify the place of bariatric surgery as a long-term treatment for type 2 diabetes, which should include data on the acceptability of bariatric surgery compared with other approaches to treating diabetes. Advances in surgical techniques have significantly reduced the risk for overall peri-operative mortality to less than 1% in experienced hands, but the surgery can cause a variety of complications, including electrolyte abnormalities, nutrient deficiencies, kidney stones, and osteoporosis. Long-term micronutrient replacement and life-long follow-up are therefore required. Furthermore, the procedures have a major impact on the way a person eats, emphasizing the need to address the psychological effects of bariatric surgery as well as a clear explanation of risks and complication rates in any patients considering this option. Given the expense, potential hazards and need for long-term patient management, bariatric surgery should not be considered lightly as a primary treatment for diabetes. It should also be noted that remission of diabetes or improvements in the condition are not seen in all patients, implying that those with certain characteristics derive most benefit. Much research is still required into the mechanisms of diabetes remission following bariatric surgery, which in the long term may lead to the development of non-surgical methods with the same effects.

References

Buchwald H, Estok R, Fahrbach K, *et al.* (2009) Weight and type 2 diabetes after bariatric surgery: systematic review and meta-analysis. *Am J Med*; 122:248–256.

Kopelman P. (2010) Symposium 1: Overnutrition: consequences and solutions. Foresight Report: the obesity challenge ahead. *Proc Nutr Soc*; 69:80–85.

National Institute for Health and Clinical Excellence (NICE) (2006) Obesity: the prevention, identification, assessment and management of overweight and obesity in adults and children. Available from: www.nice.org.uk/guidance/CG43. Last accessed February 2010.

Pinkney JH, Kerrigan D. (2004) Current status of bariatric surgery in the treatment of type 2 diabetes. *Obesity Reviews*; 5:69–78.

Rubino F, Kaplan LM, Schauer PR, Cummings DE; On Behalf of the Diabetes Surgery Summit Delegates (2009) The Diabetes Surgery Summit Consensus Conference: Recommendations for the evaluation and use of gastrointestinal surgery to treat type 2 diabetes mellitus. *Ann Surg*; 251:399–405.

Rubino F, R'bibo SL, del Genio F, *et al.* (2010) Metabolic surgery: the role of the gastrointestinal tract in diabetes mellitus. *Nat Rev Endocrinol*; 6:102–109.

Vetter ML, Cardillo S, Rickels MR, Iqbal N. (2009) Narrative review: effect of bariatric surgery on type 2 diabetes mellitus. *Ann Intern Med*; 150:94–103.

9   Organization of Diabetes Care

Diabetes is a chronic illness that requires continuing medical care and patient education to prevent acute complications and to reduce the risk of long-term morbidity and mortality. The care is complex and requires that many issues, beyond glycaemic control, are addressed. As a result people with diabetes form a significant part of the workload of healthcare providers and an estimated 10% of the entire National Health Service (NHS) budget (Baxter *et al.*, 2006).

As outlined by the Management Of Diabetes for ExceLlence (MODEL) group, a national model of care is required that can increase the capacity of the healthcare system as a whole to meet the needs of the growing number of people with diabetes, with care provided in the right place at the right time and with the right amount of expertise (Vanterpool, 2008).

There is increasing emphasis for diabetes to be managed in primary care; NHS Diabetes, formerly the National Diabetes Support Team, state that approximately 80% of diabetes care can be delivered in this setting. The level of responsibility for diabetes care expected by government from primary care providers has been formalized through service frameworks, which lay down the minimum standards for the prevention, diagnosis and management of diabetes, and by the Quality and Outcomes Framework targets for diabetes care set out in the General Medical Services contract. However, although a high level of care is delivered by many practices, there remains inequality with much higher rates of diabetes in some deprived areas of the UK compared with the national average. To provide effective diabetes care for all, ways of maximizing capacity at a local level are required.

Managing diabetes in primary care

For many people with diabetes, their GP and practice nurse, who has often completed extra training in diabetes care and does much of the routine checking and health promotion, will provide most of the help and advice they need. They will also have access to an expanded primary care team, which will include a podiatrist, dietician and optometrist. A key member of the

New Mechanisms in Glucose Control, First Edition. Anthony H. Barnett & Jenny Grice.
© 2011 Anthony H. Barnett & Jenny Grice. Published 2011 Blackwell Publishing Ltd.

> ### Box 9.1 Examples of services that can be delivered by diabetes specialist nurses
>
> • Education and skill development so individuals with diabetes can manage their condition to the best of their ability.
> • Specialist advice and support to individuals with diabetes.
> • Education, advice and support to professional and non-professional staff, who care for people with diabetes.
> • Group education for people starting on insulin or changing their insulin.
> • Crisis management advice and support for people with diabetes or their carers (such as at times of illness and hypoglycaemia).

multidisciplinary diabetes team is the diabetes specialist nurse whose role has expanded and developed to meet the needs of the ever-growing diabetes population and government directives (Box 9.1). The patient with diabetes has many different learning needs relating to diet, monitoring and treatments. Diabetes specialist nurses provide many of these needs, aiming to help people self-manage their condition. Diabetes specialist nurses generally cover a primary care trust, but work closely with primary care teams. Effective use of specialist nursing provides the patient with a constant point of contact and saves on valuable GP time.

Ethnic minorities such as South Asians can often miss out on diabetes care due to language and cultural barriers, even though they are often those with the greatest need because of a higher prevalence of diabetes in this population (Barnett *et al.*, 2006). In areas with large populations of South Asians, a successful introduction has been the use of link workers, who speak the language and understand the culture of particular South Asian groups (Bellary *et al.*, 2008; O'Hare *et al.*, 2004). Link workers help break down barriers and improve access to information and diabetes services. Working with nurses, they can perform many of the routine tasks involved in diabetes health reviews such as blood pressure monitoring and blood taking, explaining what the tests are for in the language the patient understands. In some primary care trusts, link workers also run education sessions in the Asian community for people with diabetes, offering simple lifestyle advice, healthy cooking techniques, and information on how to manage diabetes during Ramadan.

Delivery of diabetes care closer to home

Organizing diabetes care so that it can be provided closer to a patient's home or place of work is more convenient for patients and reduces non-attendance, which in turn benefits the NHS – missed appointments are costly to the health service and deprive other patients of consultant time. The development of community diabetes clinics has been an important step in achieving this. The clinics allow people with newly diagnosed diabetes and those needing treatment adjustments to see a healthcare provider, often a diabetes specialist nurse, immediately without the need for referral to specialist care. Patients attending diabetes clinics receive the same quality of care that they would in a hospital, but the location of the clinic in the community means that patients should not have so far to travel.

Structured patient education programmes

It is estimated that on average a person with diabetes spends only three hours a year with a health professional; the rest of the time they must manage the condition themselves. Self-management skills are therefore essential for good diabetes care and will include understanding and making decisions about their medication, diet and physical activity. To help patients achieve this the National Service Framework for diabetes states that all primary care trusts must commit to offering structured education programmes to people with type 2 diabetes from the point of diagnosis and as an ongoing part of their therapy in the long term. Diabetes Education and Self-management for Ongoing and Newly Diagnosed (DESMOND) is such a structured education programme designed for patients with type 2 diabetes, and is the first one to meet the criteria set down by the National Institute for Health and Clinical Excellence (NICE) for suitable education programmes (NICE, 2003). The effectiveness of the programme has been evaluated in a randomized controlled trial. Both the DESMOND and usual care arms demonstrated reductions in HbA_{1c}, although there was no significant difference between the two (Davies *et al.*, 2008). Compared with no structured education, DESMOND was associated with benefits on illness beliefs, weight loss, physical activity, smoking status and depression, which were sustained over 12 months from diagnosis.

Improving community services for those with diabetes is a priority issue. By moving the focus of diabetes services out of hospital and into the local community care is being designed around patients' needs with the aim of reducing health inequalities and ultimately morbidity and mortality rates.

References

Barnett AH, Dixon AN, Bellary S, *et al.* (2006) Type 2 diabetes and cardiovascular risk in the UK south Asian community. *Diabetologia*; 49:2234–2246.

Baxter M, Gadsby R, Griffiths U, Baxter M. (2006) Empowering primary care practitioners to meet the growing challenge of diabetes care in the community. *Br J Diabetes Vasc Dis*; 6:245–248.

Bellary S, O'Hare JP, Raymond NT, *et al.*; UKADS Study Group (2008) Enhanced diabetes care to patients of south Asian ethnic origin (the United Kingdom Asian Diabetes Study): a cluster randomised controlled trial. *Lancet*; 371:1769–1776.

Davies MJ, Heller S, Skinner TC, *et al.*; Diabetes Education and Self Management for Ongoing and Newly Diagnosed Collaborative (2008) Effectiveness of the diabetes education and self management for ongoing and newly diagnosed (DESMOND) programme for people with newly diagnosed type 2 diabetes: cluster randomised controlled trial. *BMJ*; 336:491–495.

National Institute for Health and Clinical Excellence (NICE) (2003) Diabetes (types 1 and 2) – patient education models (No. 60): The clinical effectiveness and cost effectiveness of patient education models for diabetes (April 2003). Available from: http://www.nice.org.uk/page.aspx?o=TA060. Last accessed February 2010.

O'Hare JP, Raymond NT, Mughal S, *et al.*; UKADS Study Group (2004) Evaluation of delivery of enhanced diabetes care to patients of South Asian ethnicity: the United Kingdom Asian Diabetes Study (UKADS). *Diabet Med*; 21:1357–1365.

Vanterpool G. (2008) Working together for excellence in diabetes. *Practice Nursing*; 19:20–22.

Index

Page numbers in *italics* denote figures and tables.

New Mechanisms in Glucose Control, First Edition. Anthony H. Barnett & Jenny Grice.
© 2011 Anthony H. Barnett & Jenny Grice. Published 2011 Blackwell Publishing Ltd.